Welcome to the ***"Diabetic Cookbook for Men: 110+ Recipes to Balance Blood Sugar and Satisfy Cravings."*** *This book is your go-to resource for delicious, nutritious meals designed specifically to help men manage their diabetes effectively while enjoying flavorful dishes.*

Living with diabetes requires careful attention to what you eat, but that doesn't mean you have to compromise on taste or satisfaction. In this cookbook, you'll discover a diverse range of recipes crafted to support balanced blood sugar levels and fulfill your cravings for hearty, comforting meals. From breakfasts that kickstart your day with energy to dinners that bring families together around the table, each recipe is thoughtfully created to provide essential nutrients without sacrificing flavor.

Whether you're newly diagnosed or have been managing diabetes for years, this book offers more than just recipes. It's a comprehensive guide to healthier eating habits tailored specifically for men. You'll find practical tips on portion control, ingredient selection, and meal planning, all aimed at making it easier to integrate diabetes management into your daily life.

We understand that maintaining a healthy diet can sometimes feel challenging, especially when faced with cravings or time constraints. That's why every recipe in this book is designed to be straightforward and easy to prepare, ensuring that you can enjoy delicious meals without spending hours in the kitchen.

With over 110 recipes to explore, ranging from quick and easy snacks to satisfying main courses and decadent desserts, this cookbook is your companion on the journey to better health. Let's embark together on a flavorful adventure that proves living with diabetes doesn't mean giving up on taste or enjoyment. Here's to balanced blood sugar, satisfied cravings, and a healthier, happier you!

1. Vegetable Omelet

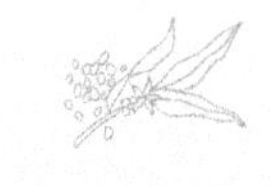

PREP TIME
20 MINUTES

COOK TIME
30 MINUTES

INGREDIENTS:

- 3 large eggs
- 2 tbsp low-fat milk
- 1/4 tsp salt
- 1/4 tsp black pepper
- 1 tsp olive oil
- 1/2 cup diced bell peppers
- 1/2 cup diced onions
- 1/2 cup diced mushrooms
- 2 tbsp shredded low-fat cheddar cheese

PROCEDURE:

1. In a small bowl, whisk together the eggs, milk, salt, and pepper until well combined.

2. Heat the olive oil in a non-stick skillet over medium heat.

3. Add the diced bell peppers, onions, and mushrooms to the skillet. Sauté for 3-4 minutes until the vegetables are tender.

4. Pour the egg mixture over the vegetables in the skillet.

5. As the eggs start to set, use a spatula to gently lift the edges, allowing the uncooked egg to flow underneath.

6. When the eggs are mostly set but still a bit soft on top, sprinkle the shredded cheddar cheese over the top.

7. Fold the omelet in half and slide it onto a plate.

This omelet is high in protein, low in carbs, and the vegetables provide fiber and important nutrients. The low-fat cheese keeps it diabetes-friendly. Enjoy!

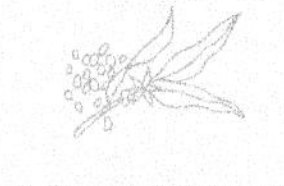

2. Greek Yogurt with Berries

PREP TIME
20 MINUTES

COOK TIME
30 MINUTES

INGREDIENTS :

- 1 cup plain, unsweetened Greek yogurt
- 1/2 cup fresh or frozen mixed berries (such as blueberries, raspberries, blackberries)
- 1 tsp honey (optional)
- 1 tbsp chopped walnuts or sliced almonds (optional)

PROCEDURE :

1. Spoon the Greek yogurt into a serving bowl or container.

2. Top the yogurt with the mixed berries.

3. If desired, drizzle the honey over the top of the berries.

4. Sprinkle the chopped nuts over the top.

That's it! This makes a quick, easy, and nutritious breakfast or snack.

The Greek yogurt provides protein, calcium, and probiotics. The berries are full of antioxidants, fiber, and natural sweetness. The honey (if using) adds a touch of sweetness, and the nuts provide healthy fats and crunch.

This is an excellent option for men with diabetes as it is low in carbs, high in protein and fiber, and can help regulate blood sugar levels. Feel free to adjust the amounts of each ingredient to suit your personal taste preferences.

3. Chia Seed Pudding

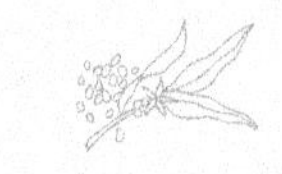 

PREP TIME
20 MINUTES

COOK TIME
30 MINUTES

INGREDIENTS :

- 1/4 cup chia seeds
- 1 cup unsweetened almond milk (or other non-dairy milk)
- 1 tsp vanilla extract
- 1/2 tsp ground cinnamon
- 1-2 tsp liquid stevia or 1 tbsp honey (optional, to taste)
- 1/4 cup fresh or frozen berries (such as blueberries, raspberries, or strawberries)
- 2 tbsp chopped nuts (such as almonds, walnuts, or pecans)

PROCEDURE :

1. In a medium bowl, whisk together the chia seeds, almond milk, vanilla, and cinnamon until well combined.

2. If using sweetener, stir in the stevia or honey now.

3. Cover the bowl and refrigerate for at least 2 hours, or overnight, stirring occasionally, until the mixture has thickened to a pudding-like consistency.

4. When ready to serve, spoon the chia pudding into bowls or jars.

5. Top each serving with 2-3 tablespoons of fresh or frozen berries and 1 tablespoon of chopped nuts.

This chia seed pudding is packed with fiber, protein, healthy fats, and antioxidants - all important for managing diabetes. The chia seeds and nuts provide satisfying texture and crunch. Feel free to adjust the sweetener to your taste preferences.

This makes a great breakfast, snack, or even a light dessert for men with diabetes. It's easy to prepare ahead of time for a quick, nutritious option.

4. Avocado Toast on Whole Grain Bread

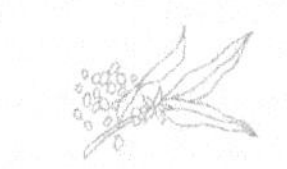

PREP TIME
20 MINUTES

COOK TIME
30 MINUTES

INGREDIENTS:

- 2 slices of whole grain or sprouted bread
- 1 medium ripe avocado, mashed
- 1 tbsp lemon juice
- 1/4 tsp salt
- 1/4 tsp black pepper
- 1 tbsp crumbled feta cheese (optional)
- 1 tbsp chopped fresh herbs (such as cilantro, basil, or chives) (optional)

PROCEDURE:

1. Toast the whole grain bread slices until lightly golden brown.

2. In a small bowl, mash the avocado with the lemon juice, salt, and black pepper until smooth and creamy.

3. Spread the mashed avocado evenly over the toasted bread slices.

4. If using, sprinkle the crumbled feta cheese and chopped fresh herbs over the top of the avocado toast.

This avocado toast makes a nutritious and satisfying breakfast or snack for men with diabetes. The whole grain bread provides complex carbs, fiber, and nutrients. The avocado is full of healthy monounsaturated fats, fiber, and vitamins. The optional feta cheese adds a boost of protein.

This recipe is easy to customize - you can add a fried or poached egg on top for extra protein, or sprinkle on some crushed red pepper flakes for a little kick. Enjoy this tasty and diabetes-friendly avocado toast!

5. Overnight Oats with Almond Milk

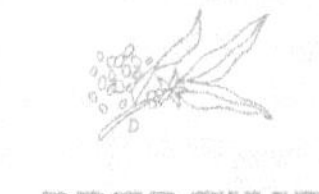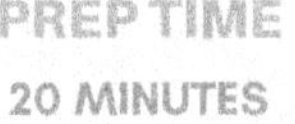

PREP TIME
20 MINUTES

COOK TIME
30 MINUTES

INGREDIENTS:

- 1/2 cup old-fashioned rolled oats
- 1 cup unsweetened almond milk
- 1 tbsp chia seeds
- 1 tsp ground cinnamon
- 1/2 tsp vanilla extract
- 1-2 tsp liquid stevia or 1 tbsp honey (optional, to taste)
- 1/4 cup fresh or frozen berries (such as blueberries, raspberries, or strawberries)
- 2 tbsp chopped nuts (such as almonds, walnuts, or pecans)

PROCEDURE:

1. In a medium bowl or mason jar, combine the rolled oats, almond milk, chia seeds, cinnamon, and vanilla extract.

2. If using a sweetener, stir it in now.

3. Cover and refrigerate the mixture overnight, or for at least 4-6 hours.

4. When ready to serve, top the overnight oats with the fresh or frozen berries and chopped nuts.

This overnight oats recipe is perfect for men with diabetes. The oats provide complex carbs, fiber, and protein to help regulate blood sugar levels. The almond milk is low in carbs and high in healthy fats. The chia seeds add extra fiber, protein, and omega-3s.

You can adjust the sweetener to your taste preferences - the berries provide natural sweetness as well. The nuts add a satisfying crunch and healthy fats.

This make-ahead breakfast is easy, nutritious, and delicious. Enjoy it chilled or at room temperature. It's a great option for busy mornings or to meal prep for the week.

6. Scrambled Tofu with Vegetables

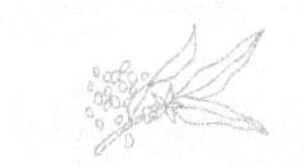

PREP TIME
20 MINUTES

COOK TIME
30 MINUTES

INGREDIENTS:

- 1 block (14 oz) firm or extra-firm tofu, drained and crumbled
- 1 tbsp olive oil
- 1/2 cup diced onions
- 1/2 cup diced bell peppers
- 1/2 cup sliced mushrooms
- 2 cloves garlic, minced
- 1 tsp ground turmeric
- 1/2 tsp ground cumin
- 1/4 tsp salt
- 1/4 tsp black pepper
- 2 tbsp chopped fresh parsley or cilantro (optional)

PROCEDURE:

1. Heat the olive oil in a large non-stick skillet over medium heat.

2. Add the diced onions, bell peppers, and mushrooms. Sauté for 5-7 minutes until the vegetables are tender.

3. Add the minced garlic and sauté for 1 minute until fragrant.

4. Crumble the tofu into the skillet and stir to combine with the vegetables.

5. Sprinkle in the turmeric, cumin, salt, and black pepper. Stir to coat the tofu and vegetables evenly.

6. Cook for 5-7 minutes, stirring occasionally, until the tofu is heated through and the flavors have melded.

7. Remove from heat and stir in the chopped parsley or cilantro, if using.

Serve the scrambled tofu warm, on its own or with a side of whole grain toast or roasted potatoes. This dish is high in protein, low in carbs, and packed with fiber and nutrients from the vegetables.

The turmeric and cumin add great flavor and anti-inflammatory benefits. This makes a satisfying and diabetes-friendly breakfast or brunch option for men.

7. Cottage Cheese with Fresh Fruit

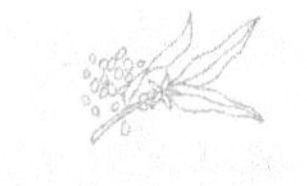

PREP TIME
20 MINUTES

COOK TIME
30 MINUTES

INGREDIENTS :

- 1 cup low-fat or non-fat cottage cheese
- 1 cup mixed fresh fruit (such as berries, diced apple, diced mango, etc.)
- 1 tsp honey (optional)
- Cinnamon (optional)

PROCEDURE :

1. Scoop the cottage cheese into a bowl or container.

2. Top the cottage cheese with the mixed fresh fruit.

3. If desired, drizzle the honey over the top.

4. Sprinkle a light dusting of cinnamon over the fruit and cottage cheese (optional).

That's it! This makes a quick, easy, and nutritious snack or light meal

8. Smoothie with Spinach, Berries, and Protein Powder

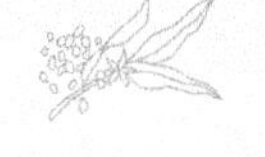 

PREP TIME
20 MINUTES

COOK TIME
30 MINUTES

INGREDIENTS :

- 1 cup unsweetened almond milk (or other non-dairy milk)
- 1 cup fresh spinach leaves
- 1 cup frozen mixed berries (such as blueberries, raspberries, strawberries)
- 1 scoop vanilla or unflavored protein powder (about 20-25g protein)
- 1 tbsp ground flaxseed
- 1 tsp honey (optional)
- Ice cubes (as needed)

PROCEDURE :

1. Add the almond milk, spinach, frozen berries, protein powder, and flaxseed to a high-powered blender.

2. Blend on high speed until the mixture is smooth and creamy, about 1-2 minutes.

3. If using honey, add it now and blend briefly to incorporate.

4. Add ice cubes as needed to reach your desired thickness and consistency.

5. Pour the smoothie into a glass and enjoy immediately.

This smoothie is packed with nutrients that are great for managing diabetes:

- Spinach provides fiber, vitamins, and antioxidants
- Berries are low in sugar and high in fiber, vitamins, and antioxidants
- Protein powder helps stabilize blood sugar and keeps you feeling full
- Flaxseed adds healthy omega-3 fats and more fiber

The almond milk keeps the carb count low, and the honey (if using) provides a touch of natural sweetness.

This makes a nutritious and satisfying breakfast, snack, or post-workout recovery drink for men with diabetes. Feel free to adjust the ingredients to your taste preferences.

9. Quinoa Breakfast Bowl

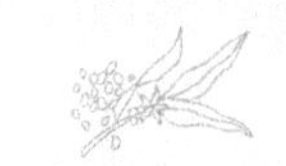

PREP TIME
20 MINUTES

COOK TIME
30 MINUTES

INGREDIENTS :

- 1/2 cup cooked quinoa, cooled
- 1/2 cup unsweetened almond milk
- 1 tbsp chia seeds
- 1 tsp ground cinnamon
- 1/4 tsp vanilla extract
- 1-2 tsp honey or maple syrup (optional)
- 1/4 cup fresh berries (such as blueberries, raspberries, or sliced strawberries)
- 2 tbsp chopped walnuts or almonds

PROCEDURE :

1. In a medium bowl, combine the cooked quinoa, almond milk, chia seeds, cinnamon, and vanilla extract. Stir well to mix.

2. If using a sweetener, drizzle the honey or maple syrup over the top and stir to incorporate.

3. Top the quinoa mixture with the fresh berries and chopped nuts.

This quinoa breakfast bowl is a great option for men with diabetes. Quinoa is a whole grain that is high in fiber, protein, and complex carbs to help regulate blood sugar levels. The chia seeds and nuts provide healthy fats and additional fiber.

The berries add natural sweetness, vitamins, and antioxidants. The almond milk keeps the carb count low compared to dairy milk.

You can adjust the sweetener to your taste preferences, or omit it entirely if the berries provide enough natural sweetness for you. This makes a satisfying and nutritious breakfast that will keep you feeling full and energized.

Feel free to experiment with different fruit and nut combinations as well. This is a very versatile and diabetes-friendly breakfast option.

10. Low-Carb Pancakes

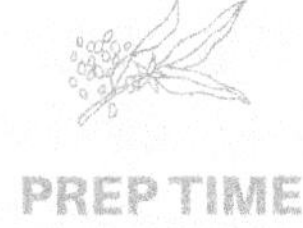

PREP TIME
20 MINUTES

COOK TIME
30 MINUTES

INGREDIENTS:

- 1/2 cup almond flour
- 2 tablespoons coconut flour
- 1 teaspoon baking powder
- 1/4 teaspoon salt
- 2 large eggs
- 1/4 cup unsweetened almond milk
- 1 tablespoon melted coconut oil or butter
- 1 teaspoon vanilla extract
- 1-2 teaspoons zero-calorie sweetener (optional)

Toppings (optional):
- Fresh berries
- Chopped nuts
- Sugar-free maple syrup
- Whipped cream

PROCEDURE:

1. In a medium bowl, whisk together the almond flour, coconut flour, baking powder, and salt.

2. In a separate bowl, beat the eggs. Then stir in the almond milk, melted coconut oil/butter, and vanilla extract.

3. Pour the wet ingredients into the dry ingredients and mix until just combined. Do not overmix.

4. Heat a non-stick skillet or griddle over medium heat. Scoop the batter onto the hot surface, using about 2-3 tablespoons per pancake.

5. Cook for 2-3 minutes per side, until golden brown. Flip carefully.

6. Serve the low-carb pancakes warm, with your desired toppings.

These pancakes are a great option for men with diabetes. The almond and coconut flours provide fiber and protein to help regulate blood sugar. The eggs and healthy fats from the coconut oil/butter also contribute to the nutritional profile.

Feel free to adjust the sweetener to your taste preferences. The berries, nuts, and sugar-free syrup make tasty, diabetes-friendly toppings.

Enjoy these fluffy, low-carb pancakes as part of a balanced breakfast or brunch. They're sure to satisfy your cravings while keeping your blood sugar in check.

11. Apple Slices with Peanut Butter

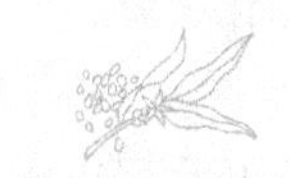

PREP TIME
20 MINUTES

COOK TIME
30 MINUTES

INGREDIENTS :

- 1 medium apple, cored and sliced into wedges
- 2 tablespoons natural peanut butter (no added sugar)

PROCEDURE :

1. Wash and slice the apple into wedges or slices.

2. Scoop the peanut butter into a small bowl or dish.

3. Dip the apple slices into the peanut butter, coating them evenly.

That's it! This simple snack is a great option for men with diabetes.

The apple provides fiber, vitamins, and natural sweetness, while the peanut butter adds protein and healthy fats to help stabilize blood sugar levels. The combination of the crisp apple and creamy peanut butter is both satisfying and delicious.

Be sure to choose a natural peanut butter without added sugars or oils. You can also experiment with other nut or seed butters like almond butter or sunflower seed butter.

This snack is portable, easy to prepare, and provides a nice balance of carbs, protein, and healthy fats. It makes a great pick-me-up during the day or a light dessert option.

Adjust the portion sizes as needed to fit your individual dietary needs. Enjoy this tasty and diabetes-friendly snack!

12. Mixed Nuts

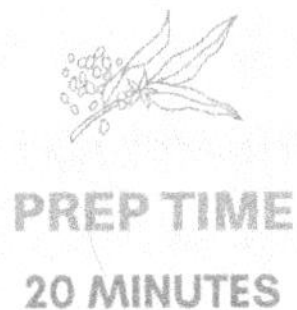

PREP TIME
20 MINUTES

COOK TIME
30 MINUTES

INGREDIENTS :

- 1/4 cup raw, unsalted almonds
- 1/4 cup raw, unsalted walnuts
- 1/4 cup raw, unsalted pecans
- 1/4 cup raw, unsalted cashews
- 1/4 tsp ground cinnamon (optional)
- 1/8 tsp sea salt (optional)

1. In a small bowl, combine the almonds, walnuts, pecans, and cashews.

2. If desired, sprinkle the cinnamon and sea salt over the nuts and toss to coat evenly.

That's it! This simple mixed nut snack is ready to enjoy.

Nuts are an excellent choice for men with diabetes. They are high in healthy fats, protein, fiber, and various vitamins and minerals. The combination of different nuts provides a variety of nutrients.

The cinnamon and salt are optional, but can add a nice flavor boost. Just be mindful of the sodium content if you have any restrictions.

This mixed nut snack is portable, shelf-stable, and satisfying. The healthy fats and protein help keep blood sugar levels stable and provide lasting energy.

Portion control is key, as nuts are calorie-dense. Stick to the 1/4 cup serving size recommended. You can also try mixing in some seeds like pumpkin or sunflower seeds for extra variety.

This makes a great snack on its own or paired with fresh fruit. Enjoy this diabetic-friendly mixed nut option!

13. Celery Sticks with Hummus

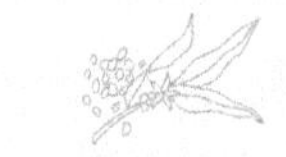

PREP TIME
20 MINUTES

COOK TIME
30 MINUTES

INGREDIENTS :

- 3-4 stalks of celery, cut into 4-inch sticks
- 1/2 cup of store-bought or homemade hummus

PROCEDURE :

1. Wash the celery stalks and cut them into 4-inch sticks.

2. Scoop the hummus into a small serving bowl or dish.

3. Arrange the celery sticks around the hummus, using them as "dippers".

That's it! This simple snack is perfect for men with diabetes.

The celery provides a crunchy, low-carb vehicle for the hummus. Hummus is made from chickpeas, which are high in fiber and protein to help regulate blood sugar levels.

The combination of the fiber-rich celery and protein-packed hummus makes this a satisfying and nutritious snack. It's also easy to prepare and portable, making it great for on-the-go.

You can use any variety of hummus you enjoy - classic, roasted red pepper, garlic, or even a lower-fat version. Just be sure to check the nutrition label and choose a hummus without added sugars.

This makes a great afternoon pick-me-up or a healthy side to pair with a meal. Feel free to adjust the portion sizes to fit your individual dietary needs.

14. Hard-Boiled Eggs

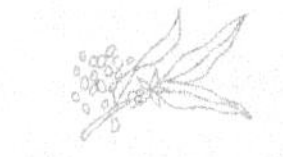

PREP TIME
20 MINUTES

COOK TIME
30 MINUTES

INGREDIENTS:

- 6 large eggs

PROCEDURE:

1. Place the eggs in a single layer in a saucepan and cover with cold water by 1 inch.

2. Bring the water to a boil over high heat. Once the water reaches a full boil, remove the pan from the heat and cover.

3. Let the eggs sit in the hot water for the following times:
- Soft-boiled: 6-7 minutes
- Hard-boiled: 12 minutes

4. Drain the hot water and cover the eggs with cold water. Let sit for 5 minutes.

5. Peel the eggs and enjoy!

Hard-boiled eggs are an excellent diabetic-friendly snack for men. They are high in protein, which helps stabilize blood sugar levels, and they contain no carbs.

The protein in eggs also helps promote feelings of fullness, making this a satisfying and nutritious option. Hard-boiled eggs are also very portable and easy to prepare in advance.

You can enjoy the hard-boiled eggs on their own, or pair them with other healthy snacks like sliced vegetables, a small serving of nuts, or a piece of whole grain toast.

For added flavor, you can sprinkle the peeled eggs with a bit of salt, pepper, paprika, or other spices. Just be mindful of any sodium restrictions in your diabetes management plan.

Hard-boiled eggs are a versatile, diabetes-friendly snack that can be easily incorporated into a healthy eating plan for men. Give this simple recipe a try!

15. Cheese and Whole Grain Crackers

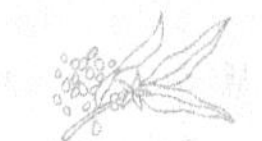 

PREP TIME
20 MINUTES

COOK TIME
30 MINUTES

INGREDIENTS :

- 1 oz (about 1-2 slices) low-fat cheddar or mozzarella cheese
- 6-8 whole grain crackers (look for ones with at least 3g fiber per serving)

PROCEDURE :

1. Slice or cube the cheese into bite-sized pieces.

2. Arrange the cheese pieces and whole grain crackers on a small plate or in a portable container.

This simple snack provides a balance of protein, fiber, and complex carbs - all important for managing diabetes.

The cheese offers protein and healthy fats to help slow the absorption of carbs from the crackers. The whole grain crackers provide fiber and complex carbohydrates, which are better for blood sugar regulation compared to refined grains.

This snack is portable, easy to prepare, and satisfying. The combination of the crunchy crackers and creamy cheese makes it a tasty option for men with diabetes.

You can experiment with different types of cheese, such as Swiss, pepper jack, or goat cheese. Just be mindful of portion sizes, as cheese can be high in calories and saturated fat.

Pair this snack with some fresh vegetables, like carrot or celery sticks, for added fiber and nutrients. This makes a great mid-afternoon pick-me-up or a light pre-workout snack.

Remember to always check nutrition labels and choose whole grain crackers with minimal added sugars or sodium.

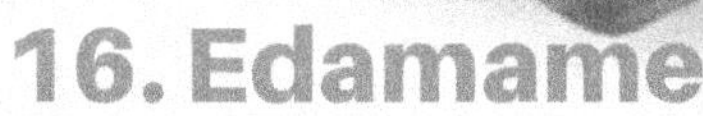

16. Edamame

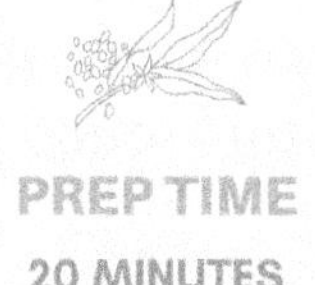

PREP TIME
20 MINUTES

COOK TIME
30 MINUTES

INGREDIENTS:

- 1 lb fresh or frozen edamame in the pod
- 1 tsp sea salt (or to taste)
- 1 tsp sesame oil (optional)

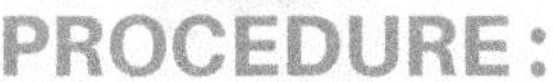

PROCEDURE:

1. If using frozen edamame, bring a large pot of water to a boil. Add the frozen edamame and cook for 5-7 minutes until tender. Drain and rinse with cold water.

2. If using fresh edamame, bring a large pot of salted water to a boil. Add the fresh edamame pods and cook for 5-7 minutes until tender. Drain and rinse with cold water.

3. Transfer the cooked edamame to a serving bowl. Sprinkle with sea salt and toss to coat evenly.

4. If desired, drizzle the sesame oil over the edamame and toss gently to coat.

Serve the edamame warm or at room temperature. You can also refrigerate leftovers for up to 3-4 days.

Edamame is an excellent snack or side dish for men with diabetes. It's high in protein, fiber, and nutrients like folate, vitamin K, and antioxidants. The fiber and protein help slow the absorption of carbs, keeping blood sugar levels stable.

The simple seasoning of just salt (and optional sesame oil) allows the natural flavors of the edamame to shine. This is a great diabetes-friendly option that's easy to prepare and enjoy.

17. Greek Yogurt with Cucumber Slices

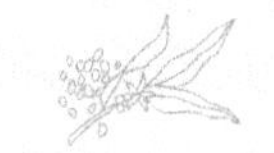 

PREP TIME
20 MINUTES

COOK TIME
30 MINUTES

INGREDIENTS:

- 1 cup plain, unsweetened Greek yogurt
- 1 medium cucumber, sliced into rounds
- 1 tbsp chopped fresh dill (optional)
- 1/4 tsp salt
- 1/4 tsp black pepper

PROCEDURE:

1. Scoop the Greek yogurt into a small bowl or container.

2. Wash and slice the cucumber into thin rounds.

3. Arrange the cucumber slices around the Greek yogurt.

4. If using, sprinkle the chopped fresh dill over the top.

5. Season with salt and black pepper.

This simple snack is a great option for men with diabetes. The Greek yogurt provides protein and probiotics, while the cucumber offers hydration, fiber, and vitamins.

The combination of the cool, crunchy cucumber and the creamy, tangy yogurt makes for a refreshing and satisfying snack. The dill adds a nice herbal flavor, but is optional.

Be sure to choose a plain, unsweetened Greek yogurt to keep the carb count low. You can also experiment with different herbs or spices to change up the flavor.

This snack is easy to prepare, portable, and provides a nice balance of nutrients to help manage blood sugar levels. Enjoy it as a mid-afternoon pick-me-up or a light side to a larger meal.

Remember to adjust the portion sizes to fit your individual dietary needs. This makes a great diabetic-friendly option for men.

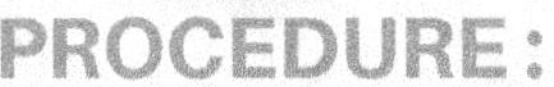

18. Kale Chips

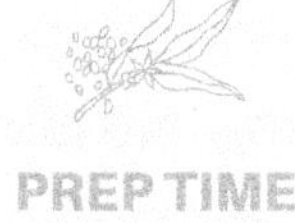

PREP TIME
20 MINUTES

COOK TIME
30 MINUTES

INGREDIENTS :

- 1 bunch of kale, washed and dried thoroughly
- 1 tbsp olive oil
- 1/4 tsp salt
- 1/4 tsp black pepper
- 1/4 tsp garlic powder (optional)

PROCEDURE :

1. Preheat your oven to 325°F (165°C).

2. Wash the kale and pat it completely dry with paper towels or a clean kitchen towel. Make sure there is no moisture left on the leaves.

3. Tear the kale leaves into bite-sized pieces, discarding any tough stems.

4. In a large bowl, toss the kale pieces with the olive oil, salt, black pepper, and garlic powder (if using) until the leaves are evenly coated.

5. Spread the kale pieces out in a single layer on a large baking sheet lined with parchment paper.

6. Bake for 12-15 minutes, flipping the kale halfway through, until the leaves are crispy and lightly browned.

7. Remove the kale chips from the oven and let cool completely before serving.

Kale chips make a great diabetic-friendly snack. Kale is low in carbs, high in fiber, and packed with vitamins, minerals, and antioxidants. The olive oil provides healthy fats to help slow the absorption of carbs.

This simple recipe allows the natural flavors of the kale to shine, with just a touch of seasoning. You can experiment with different spices and herbs to change up the flavor profile.

Kale chips are crunchy, satisfying, and much lower in calories and carbs compared to traditional potato chips. They make a great alternative for men with diabetes who are craving a salty, crispy snack.

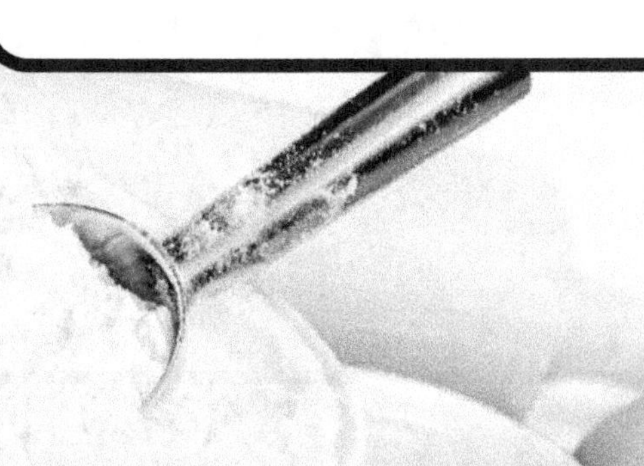

19. Sliced Bell Peppers with Guacamole

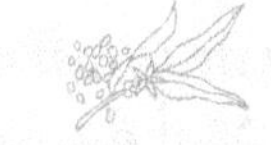 

PREP TIME
20 MINUTES

COOK TIME
30 MINUTES

INGREDIENTS:

- 1 medium avocado, mashed
- 2 tbsp diced onion
- 1 tbsp diced tomato
- 1 tsp lime juice
- 1/4 tsp salt
- 1/4 tsp ground cumin
- 1 red or yellow bell pepper, sliced into strips

PROCEDURE:

1. In a small bowl, mash the avocado with a fork until smooth.

2. Stir in the diced onion, diced tomato, lime juice, salt, and cumin. Mix well to combine.

3. Arrange the sliced bell pepper strips around the guacamole in a serving dish.

This snack is a great option for men with diabetes. The bell peppers provide fiber, vitamins, and antioxidants, while the guacamole offers healthy fats, fiber, and a creamy texture.

The guacamole is made with simple, diabetes-friendly ingredients. Avocado is high in monounsaturated fats that can help improve insulin sensitivity. The onion, tomato, lime, and spices add flavor without adding many carbs.

This snack is portable, easy to prepare, and satisfying. The crunchy bell peppers pair perfectly with the rich, flavorful guacamole.

You can adjust the amount of guacamole to suit your portion size needs. Serve this as a snack or pair it with a lean protein for a light meal.

The combination of the nutrient-dense vegetables and healthy fats makes this a great diabetic-friendly option for men. Enjoy this tasty and nutritious snack!

20. Almond Butter on Whole Grain Crackers

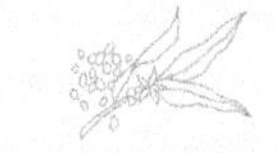

PREP TIME
20 MINUTES

COOK TIME
30 MINUTES

INGREDIENTS:

- 2 tablespoons natural almond butter (no added sugar)
- 6-8 whole grain crackers

PROCEDURE:

1. Spread the almond butter evenly over the whole grain crackers.

That's it! This simple snack is ready to enjoy.

The almond butter provides healthy fats, protein, and fiber to help stabilize blood sugar levels. Whole grain crackers are a good source of complex carbohydrates, which are better for diabetes management compared to refined grains.

This snack is portable, easy to prepare, and satisfying. The combination of the creamy almond butter and crunchy crackers makes it a tasty option.

Be sure to choose a natural almond butter without added sugars or oils. You can also experiment with other nut or seed butters like peanut butter or sunflower seed butter.

Pair this snack with some fresh fruit, like apple or banana slices, for added fiber and nutrients. This makes a great mid-afternoon pick-me-up or a light pre-workout snack.

Remember to watch your portion sizes, as nuts and nut butters can be high in calories. Stick to the 2 tablespoon serving of almond butter recommended.

This is a simple, diabetic-friendly snack that provides a balance of macronutrients to keep your blood sugar in check.

21. Grilled Chicken Caesar Salad

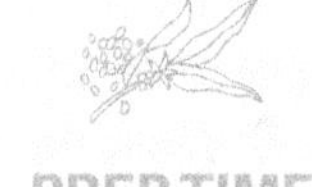

PREP TIME
20 MINUTES

COOK TIME
30 MINUTES

INGREDIENTS:

- 4 oz grilled chicken breast, sliced
- 4 cups chopped romaine lettuce
- 2 tbsp grated Parmesan cheese
- 2 tbsp low-fat Caesar dressing
- 1 tbsp toasted whole wheat croutons
- 1 tbsp sliced grilled lemon (optional)

PROCEDURE:

1. Grill or bake the chicken breast until cooked through. Slice the chicken into strips.

2. In a large salad bowl, combine the chopped romaine lettuce, grilled chicken strips, Parmesan cheese, and croutons.

3. Drizzle the low-fat Caesar dressing over the salad and toss gently to coat.

4. If desired, garnish the salad with a few slices of grilled lemon.

This grilled chicken Caesar salad is a great option for men with diabetes. The romaine lettuce provides fiber, vitamins, and minerals, while the grilled chicken adds lean protein to help stabilize blood sugar levels.

The Parmesan cheese and low-fat Caesar dressing provide creaminess and flavor without too many carbs. The whole wheat croutons add a nice crunch.

Be sure to choose a low-fat or reduced-sugar Caesar dressing to keep the carb and calorie counts in check. You can also make your own healthier Caesar dressing at home.

The grilled lemon slices are optional, but they add a nice brightness and acidity to balance the richness of the salad.

This salad makes a satisfying and diabetes-friendly main dish. You can also serve it as a side salad to accompany a lean protein like grilled fish or steak.

Adjust the portion sizes as needed to fit your individual dietary requirements. Enjoy this tasty and nutritious grilled chicken Caesar salad!

22. Spinach Salad with Walnuts and Goat Cheese

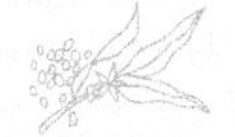 

PREP TIME
20 MINUTES

COOK TIME
30 MINUTES

INGREDIENTS:

- 5 cups fresh spinach leaves, washed and dried
- 1/4 cup crumbled goat cheese
- 2 tbsp chopped walnuts
- 1 tbsp olive oil
- 1 tbsp balsamic vinegar
- 1 tsp Dijon mustard
- 1 tsp honey (optional)
- 1/4 tsp salt
- 1/4 tsp black pepper

PROCEDURE:

1. In a large salad bowl, combine the fresh spinach leaves, crumbled goat cheese, and chopped walnuts.

2. In a small bowl, whisk together the olive oil, balsamic vinegar, Dijon mustard, honey (if using), salt, and black pepper to make the dressing.

3. Drizzle the dressing over the spinach salad and toss gently to coat.

This spinach salad is an excellent option for men with diabetes. Spinach is packed with vitamins, minerals, and antioxidants, while providing very few carbs. The walnuts add healthy fats and protein to help stabilize blood sugar levels.

The creamy goat cheese provides a nice contrast to the greens and nuts. The simple balsamic vinaigrette dressing is low in carbs and adds a tangy flavor.

The honey in the dressing is optional - the salad will still be delicious without it. You can also experiment with different nuts, such as pecans or almonds, if desired.

This salad makes a great lunch or light dinner. It's easy to prepare and very portable, making it a convenient option for busy men with diabetes.

Pair this spinach salad with a lean protein, such as grilled chicken or salmon, for a complete and diabetes-friendly meal. Enjoy!

23. Greek Salad with Feta and Olives

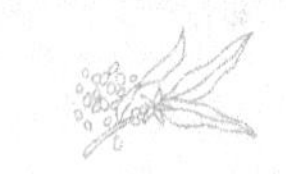

PREP TIME
20 MINUTES

COOK TIME
30 MINUTES

INGREDIENTS :

- 4 cups chopped romaine lettuce
- 1 cup diced cucumber
- 1/2 cup diced tomatoes
- 1/4 cup sliced kalamata olives
- 2 tbsp crumbled feta cheese
- 1 tbsp red wine vinegar
- 1 tbsp olive oil
- 1 tsp dried oregano
- 1/4 tsp salt
- 1/4 tsp black pepper

PROCEDURE :

1. In a large salad bowl, combine the chopped romaine, diced cucumber, diced tomatoes, and sliced kalamata olives.

2. Sprinkle the crumbled feta cheese over the top of the salad.

3. In a small bowl, whisk together the red wine vinegar, olive oil, dried oregano, salt, and black pepper.

4. Drizzle the vinaigrette over the salad and toss gently to coat.

This Greek salad is a great option for men with diabetes. The leafy greens, vegetables, and olives provide fiber, vitamins, and antioxidants. The feta cheese adds protein and healthy fats.

The simple vinaigrette dressing is low in carbs and adds a tangy, flavorful element to the salad. You can adjust the amounts of each ingredient to suit your taste preferences.

This salad makes a refreshing and satisfying lunch or side dish. It's also easy to prepare ahead of time and pack for work or on-the-go.

Pair this Greek salad with a lean protein like grilled chicken or fish for a complete, diabetes-friendly meal. Enjoy!

24. Quinoa and Black Bean Salad

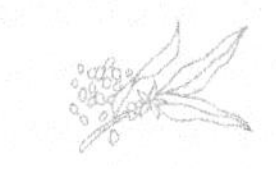 

PREP TIME
20 MINUTES

COOK TIME
30 MINUTES

INGREDIENTS:

- 1 cup cooked quinoa, cooled
- 1 (15 oz) can black beans, rinsed and drained
- 1 cup diced cucumber
- 1/2 cup diced tomatoes
- 1/4 cup diced red onion
- 2 tbsp chopped cilantro
- 2 tbsp lime juice
- 1 tbsp olive oil
- 1/2 tsp ground cumin
- 1/4 tsp salt
- 1/4 tsp black pepper

PROCEDURE:

1. In a large bowl, combine the cooked quinoa, black beans, diced cucumber, tomatoes, red onion, and chopped cilantro.

2. In a small bowl, whisk together the lime juice, olive oil, cumin, salt, and black pepper to make the dressing.

3. Pour the dressing over the quinoa and black bean salad, and toss gently to coat.

This quinoa and black bean salad is an excellent choice for men with diabetes. Quinoa is a whole grain that is high in fiber and protein, which can help regulate blood sugar levels. Black beans are also a great source of fiber and plant-based protein.

The fresh vegetables add vitamins, minerals, and antioxidants, while the lime juice and olive oil dressing provides healthy fats and a tangy flavor.

This salad is easy to prepare and can be made ahead of time for a quick, nutritious lunch or side dish. It's also very versatile - you can add other vegetables like bell peppers or corn, or swap the cilantro for parsley if desired.

The combination of complex carbs, protein, and healthy fats makes this quinoa and black bean salad a great option for managing diabetes. Enjoy it on its own or paired with a lean protein like grilled chicken or fish.

25. Kale and Apple Salad with Lemon Vinaigrette

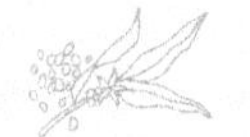

PREP TIME
20 MINUTES

COOK TIME
30 MINUTES

INGREDIENTS :

- 4 cups chopped kale, stems removed
- 1 medium apple, cored and diced
- 2 tbsp chopped walnuts
- 1 tbsp crumbled feta cheese
- 2 tbsp fresh lemon juice
- 1 tbsp olive oil
- 1 tsp Dijon mustard
- 1 tsp honey (optional)
- 1/4 tsp salt
- 1/4 tsp black pepper

PROCEDURE :

1. In a large salad bowl, combine the chopped kale, diced apple, chopped walnuts, and crumbled feta cheese.

2. In a small bowl, whisk together the lemon juice, olive oil, Dijon mustard, honey (if using), salt, and black pepper to make the vinaigrette.

3. Drizzle the lemon vinaigrette over the kale and apple salad, and toss gently to coat.

This kale and apple salad is a great option for men with diabetes. Kale is a nutrient-dense leafy green that is low in carbs and high in fiber, vitamins, and antioxidants. The apple provides natural sweetness and additional fiber.

The walnuts add healthy fats and crunch, while the feta cheese contributes protein and creaminess. The lemon vinaigrette dressing is low in carbs and provides a bright, tangy flavor.

The honey in the dressing is optional - the salad will still be delicious without it. You can also experiment with different types of apples or other nuts if desired.

This salad makes a refreshing and satisfying lunch or side dish. It's easy to prepare and the flavors pair beautifully together.

Enjoy this diabetic-friendly kale and apple salad as part of a balanced meal to help manage your blood sugar levels.

26. Cobb Salad with Turkey and Avocado

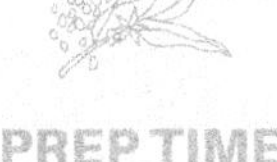

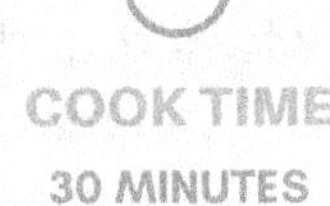

PREP TIME
20 MINUTES

COOK TIME
30 MINUTES

INGREDIENTS:

- 4 cups chopped romaine lettuce
- 3 oz cooked turkey breast, diced
- 1/2 avocado, diced
- 2 hard-boiled eggs, chopped
- 2 tbsp crumbled blue cheese
- 2 tbsp diced tomatoes
- 2 tbsp diced cucumber
- 2 tbsp low-fat ranch dressing
- 1 tbsp balsamic vinegar

PROCEDURE:

1. In a large salad bowl, arrange the chopped romaine lettuce.

2. Top the lettuce with the diced turkey breast, avocado, hard-boiled eggs, crumbled blue cheese, diced tomatoes, and diced cucumber.

3. In a small bowl, whisk together the low-fat ranch dressing and balsamic vinegar to make the dressing.

4. Drizzle the dressing over the Cobb salad and toss gently to coat.

This Cobb salad is a great option for men with diabetes. It's packed with nutrient-dense ingredients that can help regulate blood sugar levels.

The romaine lettuce, tomatoes, and cucumbers provide fiber, vitamins, and antioxidants. The turkey breast and hard-boiled eggs offer lean protein to keep you feeling full.

The avocado and blue cheese add healthy fats and creaminess to the salad. The balsamic vinegar-based dressing is low in carbs and provides a tangy flavor.

You can adjust the amounts of each ingredient to suit your personal taste preferences and dietary needs. Feel free to swap out the blue cheese for a different type of cheese, or use a different protein source like grilled chicken or shrimp.

This Cobb salad makes a satisfying and diabetes-friendly main dish or side salad. Enjoy it as part of a balanced meal to help manage your blood sugar levels.

27. Broccoli Salad with Sunflower Seeds

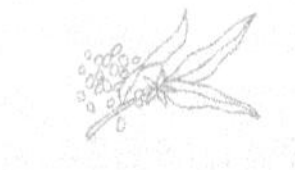 

PREP TIME
20 MINUTES

COOK TIME
30 MINUTES

INGREDIENTS :

- 4 cups chopped broccoli florets
- 2 tbsp diced red onion
- 2 tbsp unsalted sunflower seeds
- 2 tbsp plain Greek yogurt
- 1 tbsp apple cider vinegar
- 1 tsp Dijon mustard
- 1/4 tsp salt
- 1/4 tsp black pepper

PROCEDURE :

1. In a large bowl, combine the chopped broccoli florets, diced red onion, and sunflower seeds.

2. In a small bowl, whisk together the Greek yogurt, apple cider vinegar, Dijon mustard, salt, and black pepper to make the dressing.

3. Pour the dressing over the broccoli salad and toss gently to coat.

This broccoli salad is a great option for men with diabetes. Broccoli is low in carbs, high in fiber, and packed with vitamins and antioxidants. The sunflower seeds provide healthy fats and a satisfying crunch.

The Greek yogurt-based dressing adds protein and creaminess without too many carbs. The apple cider vinegar provides a tangy flavor that helps balance the sweetness of the broccoli.

This salad is easy to prepare and can be made ahead of time for a quick, nutritious side dish or snack. You can also add other crunchy vegetables like shredded carrots or diced celery if desired.

Be mindful of portion sizes, as the sunflower seeds are calorie-dense. Stick to the 2 tablespoon serving recommended.

This broccoli salad makes a great accompaniment to grilled chicken, fish, or a lean protein-based main dish. It's a tasty and diabetes-friendly option that the whole family can enjoy.

28. Tuna Salad with Mixed Greens

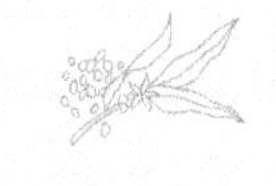 

PREP TIME
20 MINUTES

COOK TIME
30 MINUTES

INGREDIENTS :

- 1 (5 oz) can of tuna, drained and flaked
- 2 tbsp plain Greek yogurt
- 1 tbsp diced celery
- 1 tbsp diced red onion
- 1 tsp Dijon mustard
- 1 tsp lemon juice
- 1/4 tsp salt
- 1/4 tsp black pepper
- 2 cups mixed greens (such as spinach, arugula, and kale)

PROCEDURE :

1. In a medium bowl, combine the flaked tuna, Greek yogurt, diced celery, diced red onion, Dijon mustard, lemon juice, salt, and black pepper. Mix well to incorporate.

2. In a separate bowl or on a plate, arrange the 2 cups of mixed greens.

3. Top the greens with the tuna salad mixture.

This tuna salad with mixed greens is a great diabetic-friendly option for men. Tuna is an excellent source of lean protein, which can help stabilize blood sugar levels. The Greek yogurt adds creaminess and more protein without too many carbs.

The mixed greens provide fiber, vitamins, and antioxidants to round out the meal. You can use a variety of greens, such as spinach, arugula, and kale, to add different flavors and textures.

The simple dressing of Dijon mustard and lemon juice provides flavor without added sugars or oils. You can also experiment with other herbs and spices to customize the tuna salad to your taste preferences.

This makes a satisfying and nutritious lunch or light dinner. You can serve it as-is or with a side of whole grain crackers or a small portion of roasted vegetables.

Adjust the portion sizes as needed to fit your individual dietary requirements. Enjoy this diabetic-friendly tuna salad with mixed greens!

29. Roasted Beet and Arugula Salad

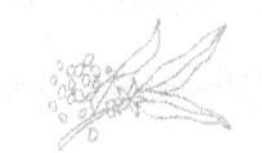

PREP TIME
20 MINUTES

COOK TIME
30 MINUTES

INGREDIENTS:

- 3 medium beets, peeled and cut into 1-inch cubes
- 1 tbsp olive oil
- 1/4 tsp salt
- 1/4 tsp black pepper
- 4 cups baby arugula
- 2 tbsp crumbled feta cheese
- 2 tbsp chopped walnuts
- 2 tbsp balsamic vinegar
- 1 tsp Dijon mustard

PROCEDURE:

1. Preheat your oven to 400°F (200°C).

2. Toss the cubed beets with the olive oil, salt, and black pepper. Spread them out in a single layer on a baking sheet.

3. Roast the beets for 25-30 minutes, stirring halfway, until they are tender and lightly caramelized.

4. Allow the roasted beets to cool slightly.

5. In a large salad bowl, combine the baby arugula, roasted beets, crumbled feta cheese, and chopped walnuts.

6. In a small bowl, whisk together the balsamic vinegar and Dijon mustard to make the dressing.

7. Drizzle the balsamic vinaigrette over the salad and toss gently to coat.

This roasted beet and arugula salad is an excellent choice for men with diabetes. Beets are low in carbs and high in fiber, vitamins, and antioxidants. Arugula is also a nutrient-dense leafy green.

The feta cheese provides protein and healthy fats, while the walnuts add crunch and more healthy fats. The balsamic vinaigrette dressing is low in carbs and adds a tangy flavor.

This salad makes a great lunch or light dinner. It's also easy to prepare in advance and pack for work or on-the-go.

Feel free to adjust the amounts of each ingredient to suit your taste preferences and dietary needs. You can also try adding other toppings like sliced avocado or grilled chicken for extra protein.

30. Chickpea and Tomato Salad

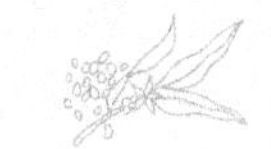

PREP TIME
20 MINUTES

COOK TIME
30 MINUTES

INGREDIENTS:

- 1 (15 oz) can chickpeas (garbanzo beans), rinsed and drained
- 1 pint cherry or grape tomatoes, halved
- 1/2 red onion, thinly sliced
- 1/4 cup fresh parsley, chopped
- 2 tbsp olive oil
- 2 tbsp red wine vinegar
- 1 tsp Dijon mustard
- 1 tsp dried oregano
- 1/4 tsp salt
- 1/4 tsp black pepper

PROCEDURE:

1. In a large bowl, combine the rinsed and drained chickpeas, halved tomatoes, sliced red onion, and chopped parsley.

2. In a small bowl, whisk together the olive oil, red wine vinegar, Dijon mustard, dried oregano, salt, and black pepper.

3. Pour the dressing over the chickpea and tomato mixture and toss gently to coat.

4. Cover and refrigerate the salad for at least 30 minutes to allow the flavors to meld.

5. Serve chilled or at room temperature.

This chickpea and tomato salad is a great option for people with diabetes. Chickpeas are a good source of fiber, protein, and complex carbohydrates, while the tomatoes provide antioxidants and vitamins. The simple dressing adds flavor without adding too many calories or carbs. This salad can be enjoyed as a main dish or a side dish.

31. Chicken Vegetable Soup

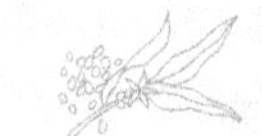

PREP TIME
20 MINUTES

COOK TIME
30 MINUTES

INGREDIENTS :

- 1 tbsp olive oil
- 1 onion, diced
- 2 carrots, peeled and diced
- 2 celery stalks, diced
- 3 cloves garlic, minced
- 1 lb boneless, skinless chicken breasts, cut into 1-inch pieces
- 6 cups low-sodium chicken broth
- 1 (15 oz) can diced tomatoes
- 1 cup frozen green beans, cut into 1-inch pieces
- 1 cup frozen peas
- 1 tsp dried thyme
- 1 tsp dried oregano
- Salt and black pepper to taste
- Fresh parsley, chopped (for garnish)

PROCEDURE :

1. In a large pot or Dutch oven, heat the olive oil over medium heat. Add the onion, carrots, and celery. Sauté for 5-7 minutes until the vegetables are softened.

2. Add the garlic and sauté for 1 minute until fragrant.

3. Add the chicken and sauté for 2-3 minutes, until the chicken is lightly browned.

4. Pour in the chicken broth, diced tomatoes, green beans, and peas. Stir to combine.

5. Add the dried thyme and oregano. Season with salt and black pepper to taste.

6. Bring the soup to a boil, then reduce the heat and let it simmer for 20-25 minutes, or until the chicken is cooked through and the vegetables are tender.

7. Serve hot, garnished with fresh chopped parsley.

This chicken vegetable soup is a great option for men with diabetes. It's low in carbs, high in protein, and packed with fiber-rich vegetables. The combination of chicken, vegetables, and herbs provides a flavorful and nutritious meal. Enjoy this comforting and diabetes-friendly soup!

32. Lentil Soup

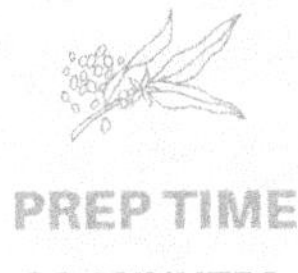

PREP TIME
20 MINUTES

COOK TIME
30 MINUTES

INGREDIENTS :

- 1 tbsp olive oil
- 1 onion, diced
- 2 carrots, peeled and diced
- 2 celery stalks, diced
- 3 cloves garlic, minced
- 1 cup dried brown or green lentils, rinsed
- 6 cups low-sodium chicken or vegetable broth
- 1 (15 oz) can diced tomatoes
- 2 tsp dried thyme
- 1 tsp dried oregano
- Salt and black pepper to taste
- Fresh parsley, chopped (for garnish)

PROCEDURE :

1. In a large pot or Dutch oven, heat the olive oil over medium heat. Add the onion, carrots, and celery. Sauté for 5-7 minutes until the vegetables are softened.

2. Add the garlic and sauté for 1 minute until fragrant.

3. Stir in the rinsed lentils, broth, diced tomatoes, thyme, and oregano. Season with salt and black pepper to taste.

4. Bring the soup to a boil, then reduce the heat and let it simmer for 25-30 minutes, or until the lentils are tender.

5. Taste and adjust seasoning as needed.

6. Serve hot, garnished with fresh chopped parsley.

This lentil soup is an excellent choice for men with diabetes. Lentils are a great source of fiber, protein, and complex carbohydrates, which can help regulate blood sugar levels. The vegetables and herbs provide additional nutrients and antioxidants. This soup is filling, satisfying, and easy to prepare, making it a great option for a healthy and diabetes-friendly meal.

33. Butternut Squash Soup

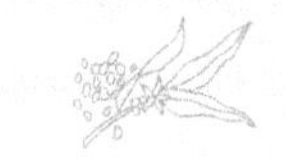

PREP TIME
20 MINUTES

COOK TIME
30 MINUTES

INGREDIENTS:

- 1 medium butternut squash, peeled, seeded, and cubed (about 4 cups)
- 1 medium onion, diced
- 2 cloves garlic, minced
- 4 cups low-sodium chicken or vegetable broth
- 1 tsp ground cinnamon
- 1/4 tsp ground nutmeg
- 1/4 tsp salt
- 1/4 tsp black pepper
- 2 tbsp plain Greek yogurt (optional garnish)
- 2 tbsp chopped fresh parsley (optional garnish)

PROCEDURE:

1. In a large pot or Dutch oven, sauté the diced onion and minced garlic in a small amount of olive oil over medium heat until softened, about 5 minutes.

2. Add the cubed butternut squash, chicken or vegetable broth, cinnamon, nutmeg, salt, and black pepper. Bring the mixture to a boil.

3. Reduce the heat to low, cover the pot, and simmer for 20-25 minutes, or until the squash is very soft.

4. Using an immersion blender or regular blender, puree the soup until smooth and creamy.

5. Serve the butternut squash soup warm, garnished with a dollop of plain Greek yogurt and chopped fresh parsley, if desired.

This butternut squash soup is an excellent option for men with diabetes. Butternut squash is low in carbs, high in fiber, and packed with vitamins and antioxidants. The cinnamon and nutmeg add warmth and flavor without any added sugars.

The Greek yogurt garnish provides a creamy texture and a boost of protein. The parsley adds a fresh, herbal note.

This soup is easy to prepare and can be made in advance for quick, nutritious meals throughout the week. It's also very versatile - you can add cooked chicken or turkey for extra protein, or serve it with a side salad or whole grain crackers.

Adjust the portion sizes as needed to fit your individual dietary requirements. Enjoy this delicious and diabetes-friendly butternut squash soup!

34. Minestrone Soup

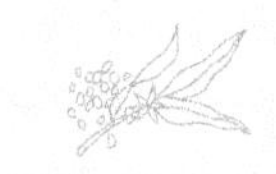

PREP TIME
20 MINUTES

COOK TIME
30 MINUTES

INGREDIENTS:

- 1 tbsp olive oil
- 1 onion, diced
- 2 carrots, peeled and diced
- 2 celery stalks, diced
- 3 cloves garlic, minced
- 1 (15 oz) can diced tomatoes
- 4 cups low-sodium chicken or vegetable broth
- 1 (15 oz) can kidney beans, rinsed and drained
- 1 (15 oz) can cannellini beans, rinsed and drained
- 1 cup frozen green beans, cut into 1-inch pieces
- 1 cup small whole wheat pasta (such as ditalini or elbow macaroni)
- 2 cups chopped kale or spinach
- 2 tsp dried Italian seasoning
- Salt and black pepper to taste
- Grated Parmesan cheese (optional)

PROCEDURE:

1. In a large pot or Dutch oven, heat the olive oil over medium heat. Add the onion, carrots, and celery. Sauté for 5-7 minutes until the vegetables are softened.

2. Add the garlic and sauté for 1 minute until fragrant.

3. Pour in the diced tomatoes, broth, kidney beans, cannellini beans, and green beans. Stir to combine.

4. Add the whole wheat pasta, kale/spinach, and Italian seasoning. Season with salt and black pepper to taste.

5. Bring the soup to a boil, then reduce the heat and let it simmer for 15-20 minutes, or until the pasta is tender.

6. Serve hot, garnished with grated Parmesan cheese if desired.

This minestrone soup is packed with fiber, protein, and nutrients, making it a great option for men with diabetes. The combination of beans, vegetables, and whole grain pasta provides a balanced and satisfying meal. Enjoy this hearty and flavorful soup!

35. Tomato Basil Soup

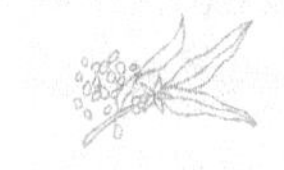 

PREP TIME
20 MINUTES

COOK TIME
30 MINUTES

INGREDIENTS:

- 1 tbsp olive oil
- 1 onion, diced
- 3 cloves garlic, minced
- 2 (14.5 oz) cans diced tomatoes
- 2 cups low-sodium chicken or vegetable broth
- 1 cup unsweetened almond milk
- 1/4 cup fresh basil, chopped
- 1 tsp dried oregano
- 1/4 tsp red pepper flakes (optional)
- Salt and black pepper to taste

PROCEDURE:

1. In a large saucepan, heat the olive oil over medium heat. Add the onion and sauté for 5-7 minutes until translucent.

2. Add the garlic and sauté for 1 minute until fragrant.

3. Pour in the diced tomatoes, broth, and almond milk. Stir to combine.

4. Add the fresh basil, oregano, and red pepper flakes (if using). Season with salt and black pepper to taste.

5. Bring the soup to a simmer and let it cook for 15-20 minutes, stirring occasionally, until the flavors have melded.

6. Using an immersion blender or regular blender, blend the soup until smooth and creamy.

7. Serve hot, garnished with additional fresh basil if desired.

This soup is low in carbs and calories, making it a great option for men with diabetes. The tomatoes provide lycopene, while the basil and garlic offer anti-inflammatory benefits. Enjoy this comforting and nutritious soup!

36. Beef and Barley Soup

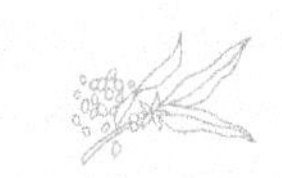

PREP TIME
20 MINUTES

COOK TIME
30 MINUTES

INGREDIENTS:

- 1 lb lean beef stew meat, cut into 1-inch cubes
- 1 tbsp olive oil
- 1 medium onion, diced
- 3 cloves garlic, minced
- 4 cups low-sodium beef broth
- 1 cup cooked pearl barley
- 2 cups diced carrots
- 2 cups diced celery
- 1 tsp dried thyme
- 1/2 tsp salt
- 1/4 tsp black pepper

PROCEDURE:

1. In a large pot or Dutch oven, heat the olive oil over medium-high heat. Add the cubed beef and brown on all sides, about 5-7 minutes. Remove the beef from the pot and set aside.

2. Add the diced onion and minced garlic to the pot. Sauté for 2-3 minutes until the onion is translucent.

3. Pour in the low-sodium beef broth and add the cooked pearl barley, diced carrots, diced celery, dried thyme, salt, and black pepper. Bring the mixture to a boil.

4. Reduce the heat to low, cover the pot, and simmer for 30-40 minutes, or until the vegetables are tender.

5. Add the browned beef back to the pot and continue simmering for an additional 10-15 minutes to allow the flavors to meld.

6. Serve the beef and barley soup hot.

This soup is a great option for men with diabetes. The lean beef provides protein, while the pearl barley adds fiber and complex carbs to help regulate blood sugar levels. The vegetables contribute vitamins, minerals, and antioxidants.

The low-sodium broth keeps the sodium content in check, and the simple seasoning of thyme, salt, and pepper allows the natural flavors to shine.

You can adjust the portion sizes to fit your individual dietary needs. This soup also freezes well, so you can make a large batch and have it on hand for quick, healthy meals.

37. Cauliflower Soup

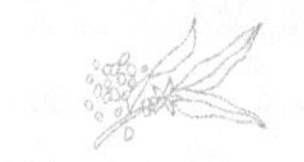

PREP TIME
20 MINUTES

COOK TIME
30 MINUTES

INGREDIENTS:

- 1 tbsp olive oil
- 1 onion, diced
- 3 cloves garlic, minced
- 1 head of cauliflower, cut into florets (about 6 cups)
- 4 cups low-sodium chicken or vegetable broth
- 1 cup unsweetened almond milk
- 1 tsp dried thyme
- 1/4 tsp ground nutmeg
- Salt and black pepper to taste
- Chopped fresh parsley for garnish (optional)

PROCEDURE:

1. In a large pot or Dutch oven, heat the olive oil over medium heat. Add the diced onion and sauté for 5-7 minutes until translucent.

2. Add the minced garlic and sauté for 1 minute until fragrant.

3. Add the cauliflower florets and the broth. Bring the mixture to a boil, then reduce the heat and let it simmer for 15-20 minutes, or until the cauliflower is very soft.

4. Using an immersion blender (or carefully transfer the soup to a regular blender), blend the soup until smooth and creamy.

5. Stir in the unsweetened almond milk, dried thyme, and ground nutmeg. Season with salt and black pepper to taste.

6. Reheat the soup if necessary, and serve hot, garnished with chopped fresh parsley if desired.

This cauliflower soup is a great option for men with diabetes. Cauliflower is low in carbs and high in fiber, which can help regulate blood sugar levels. The almond milk provides creaminess without adding too many carbs or calories. This soup is comforting, nutritious, and easy to prepare, making it a perfect diabetic-friendly meal.

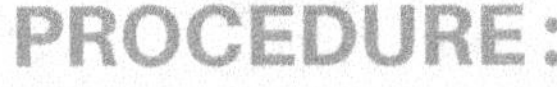

38. Split Pea Soup

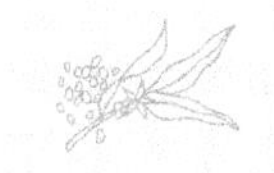

PREP TIME
20 MINUTES

COOK TIME
30 MINUTES

INGREDIENTS:

- 1 tbsp olive oil
- 1 onion, diced
- 2 carrots, peeled and diced
- 2 celery stalks, diced
- 3 cloves garlic, minced
- 1 lb dried split peas, rinsed
- 6 cups low-sodium chicken or vegetable broth
- 1 bay leaf
- 1 tsp dried thyme
- Salt and black pepper to taste
- Chopped fresh parsley for garnish (optional)

PROCEDURE:

1. In a large pot or Dutch oven, heat the olive oil over medium heat. Add the diced onion, carrots, and celery. Sauté for 5-7 minutes until the vegetables are softened.

2. Add the minced garlic and sauté for 1 minute until fragrant.

3. Stir in the rinsed split peas, broth, bay leaf, and dried thyme. Season with salt and black pepper to taste.

4. Bring the soup to a boil, then reduce the heat and let it simmer for 45-60 minutes, or until the split peas are very soft and the soup has thickened, stirring occasionally.

5. Remove the bay leaf. Using an immersion blender (or carefully transfer the soup to a regular blender), blend the soup until it reaches your desired consistency, leaving some texture if desired.

6. Taste and adjust seasoning as needed.

7. Serve hot, garnished with chopped fresh parsley if desired.

This split pea soup is an excellent choice for men with diabetes. Split peas are a great source of fiber, protein, and complex carbohydrates, which can help regulate blood sugar levels. The vegetables and herbs provide additional nutrients and antioxidants. This soup is filling, satisfying, and easy to prepare, making it a great option for a healthy and diabetes-friendly meal.

39. Zucchini and Spinach Soup

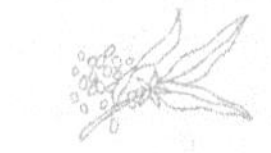

PREP TIME

20 MINUTES

COOK TIME

30 MINUTES

INGREDIENTS :

- 2 tbsp olive oil
- 1 medium onion, diced
- 3 cloves garlic, minced
- 3 medium zucchini, diced
- 4 cups low-sodium chicken or vegetable broth
- 2 cups fresh spinach leaves
- 1 tsp dried thyme
- 1/4 tsp salt
- 1/4 tsp black pepper
- 2 tbsp grated Parmesan cheese (optional garnish)

PROCEDURE :

1. In a large pot or Dutch oven, heat the olive oil over medium heat. Add the diced onion and minced garlic. Sauté for 3-4 minutes until the onion is translucent.

2. Add the diced zucchini to the pot and sauté for an additional 2-3 minutes.

3. Pour in the low-sodium broth and bring the mixture to a boil. Reduce the heat to low, cover, and simmer for 15-20 minutes, or until the zucchini is very soft.

4. Add the fresh spinach leaves and dried thyme to the pot. Stir and cook for 2-3 minutes until the spinach is wilted.

5. Using an immersion blender or regular blender, puree the soup until smooth and creamy.

6. Season the soup with salt and black pepper to taste.

7. Serve the zucchini and spinach soup warm, garnished with a sprinkle of grated Parmesan cheese if desired.

This soup is an excellent option for men with diabetes. Zucchini is low in carbs and high in fiber, while spinach provides a nutrient-dense boost of vitamins and minerals. The olive oil and Parmesan cheese (if used) add healthy fats.

The simple seasoning of thyme, salt, and pepper allows the natural flavors of the vegetables to shine. This soup is comforting, satisfying, and easy to prepare.

40. Turkey Chili

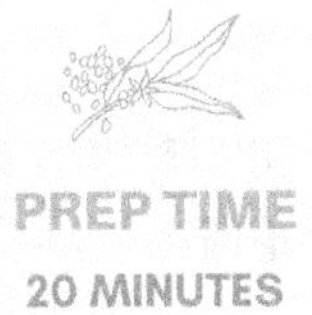 

PREP TIME
20 MINUTES

COOK TIME
30 MINUTES

INGREDIENTS:

- 1 lb ground turkey
- 1 tbsp olive oil
- 1 onion, diced
- 3 cloves garlic, minced
- 2 bell peppers, diced
- 2 (15 oz) cans diced tomatoes
- 1 (15 oz) can kidney beans, rinsed and drained
- 1 (15 oz) can black beans, rinsed and drained
- 2 tbsp chili powder
- 1 tsp ground cumin
- 1 tsp dried oregano
- 1/2 tsp smoked paprika
- 1/4 tsp cayenne pepper (optional, for heat)
- Salt and black pepper to taste
- Chopped fresh cilantro for garnish (optional)

PROCEDURE:

1. In a large pot or Dutch oven, heat the olive oil over medium-high heat. Add the ground turkey and cook, breaking it up with a wooden spoon, until it's browned and cooked through, about 5-7 minutes.

2. Add the diced onion and minced garlic to the pot. Sauté for 2-3 minutes until the onion is translucent.

3. Stir in the diced bell peppers, diced tomatoes, kidney beans, and black beans. Add the chili powder, cumin, oregano, smoked paprika, and cayenne pepper (if using). Season with salt and black pepper to taste.

4. Bring the chili to a simmer, then reduce the heat to low and let it cook for 20-25 minutes, stirring occasionally, until the flavors have melded and the chili has thickened.

5. Serve the turkey chili hot, garnished with chopped fresh cilantro if desired.

This turkey chili is a great option for men with diabetes. Ground turkey is a lean protein, and the beans provide fiber and complex carbohydrates. The vegetables and spices add flavor and antioxidants without adding too many carbs or calories. Enjoy this hearty and diabetes-friendly chili!

41. Grilled Salmon with Asparagus

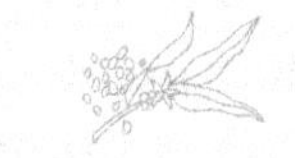 

PREP TIME
20 MINUTES

COOK TIME
30 MINUTES

INGREDIENTS:

- 4 (6 oz) salmon fillets
- 1 tbsp olive oil
- 1 tsp lemon zest
- 1 tbsp lemon juice
- 1 tsp dried dill
- 1/4 tsp salt
- 1/4 tsp black pepper
- 1 lb asparagus, trimmed
- 1 tbsp balsamic vinegar

PROCEDURE:

1. Preheat your grill or grill pan to medium-high heat.

2. In a small bowl, combine the olive oil, lemon zest, lemon juice, dried dill, salt, and black pepper. Brush this mixture over the salmon fillets.

3. Grill the salmon for 4-6 minutes per side, or until it flakes easily with a fork and reaches an internal temperature of 145°F (63°C).

4. While the salmon is grilling, place the trimmed asparagus in a grill basket or on a foil-lined grill pan. Grill the asparagus for 5-7 minutes, turning occasionally, until tender-crisp.

5. Transfer the grilled salmon and asparagus to a serving plate. Drizzle the asparagus with the balsamic vinegar.

Serve the grilled salmon and asparagus immediately, while hot.

This grilled salmon and asparagus dish is an excellent choice for men with diabetes. Salmon is a great source of lean protein and healthy omega-3 fatty acids, while asparagus is a low-carb, fiber-rich vegetable. The simple lemon-dill seasoning and balsamic vinegar add flavor without adding too many carbs or calories. This meal is both delicious and diabetes-friendly.

42. Baked Chicken with Brussels Sprouts

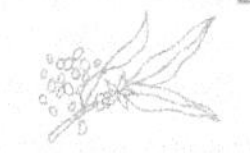

PREP TIME
20 MINUTES

COOK TIME
30 MINUTES

INGREDIENTS:

- 4 (6 oz) boneless, skinless chicken breasts
- 1 tbsp olive oil
- 1 tsp garlic powder
- 1 tsp dried thyme
- 1/2 tsp salt
- 1/4 tsp black pepper
- 1 lb Brussels sprouts, trimmed and halved
- 2 tbsp balsamic vinegar
- 1 tbsp Dijon mustard
- 1 tbsp honey

PROCEDURE:

1. Preheat your oven to 400°F (200°C).

2. In a small bowl, combine the garlic powder, dried thyme, salt, and black pepper. Rub this seasoning mixture all over the chicken breasts.

3. Heat the olive oil in a large oven-safe skillet over medium-high heat. Sear the chicken breasts on both sides until they're lightly browned, about 2-3 minutes per side.

4. Transfer the skillet to the preheated oven and bake the chicken for 15-20 minutes, or until it reaches an internal temperature of 165°F (74°C).

5. While the chicken is baking, prepare the Brussels sprouts. In a large bowl, toss the trimmed and halved Brussels sprouts with the balsamic vinegar, Dijon mustard, and honey.

6. Spread the Brussels sprouts mixture on a baking sheet and roast in the oven for 15-20 minutes, or until the sprouts are tender and lightly caramelized.

7. Serve the baked chicken with the roasted Brussels sprouts.

This baked chicken and Brussels sprouts dish is a great option for men with diabetes. The chicken is a lean protein, and the Brussels sprouts are a low-carb, fiber-rich vegetable. The balsamic-mustard glaze adds flavor without adding too many carbs or calories. Enjoy this delicious and diabetes-friendly meal!

43. Beef Stir-Fry with Vegetables

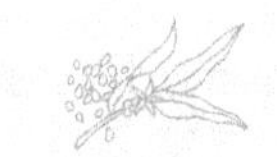

PREP TIME
20 MINUTES

COOK TIME
30 MINUTES

INGREDIENTS:

- 1 lb flank steak, thinly sliced
- 2 tbsp low-sodium soy sauce
- 1 tbsp rice vinegar
- 1 tsp sesame oil
- 1 tbsp olive oil
- 3 cloves garlic, minced
- 1 tbsp grated fresh ginger
- 1 red bell pepper, sliced
- 1 cup broccoli florets
- 1 cup snow peas or snap peas
- 1 cup sliced mushrooms
- 2 green onions, sliced
- Salt and black pepper to taste
- Cooked cauliflower rice or brown rice (optional)

PROCEDURE:

1. In a medium bowl, combine the sliced flank steak, soy sauce, rice vinegar, and sesame oil. Toss to coat the beef and let it marinate for 15-20 minutes.

2. Heat the olive oil in a large wok or skillet over high heat. Add the marinated beef and stir-fry for 2-3 minutes, until the beef is lightly browned.

3. Add the minced garlic and grated ginger to the wok and stir-fry for 1 minute until fragrant.

4. Add the sliced red bell pepper, broccoli florets, snow peas/snap peas, and sliced mushrooms to the wok. Stir-fry for 3-5 minutes, until the vegetables are tender-crisp.

5. Stir in the sliced green onions and season with salt and black pepper to taste.

6. Serve the beef and vegetable stir-fry immediately, either on its own or over a bed of cooked cauliflower rice or brown rice (if desired).

This beef stir-fry is a great option for men with diabetes. The lean beef provides protein, while the vegetables are low in carbs and high in fiber. The soy sauce, rice vinegar, and sesame oil add flavor without adding too many carbs or calories. Enjoy this delicious and diabetes-friendly meal!

44. Turkey Meatballs with Zoodles

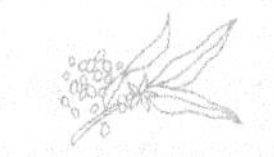 

PREP TIME
20 MINUTES

COOK TIME
30 MINUTES

INGREDIENTS:

- 1 lb ground turkey
- 1/4 cup whole wheat breadcrumbs
- 1 egg, lightly beaten
- 2 tbsp grated Parmesan cheese
- 2 cloves garlic, minced
- 1 tsp dried oregano
- 1/4 tsp salt
- 1/4 tsp black pepper
- 2 tbsp olive oil
- 3 medium zucchini, spiralized into "zoodles"
- 1 cup marinara sauce (no-sugar-added)

PROCEDURE:

1. Preheat your oven to 400°F (200°C).

2. In a large bowl, combine the ground turkey, breadcrumbs, egg, Parmesan cheese, minced garlic, dried oregano, salt, and black pepper. Mix well until the ingredients are evenly distributed.

3. Roll the turkey mixture into 1-inch meatballs and place them on a baking sheet lined with parchment paper.

4. Bake the meatballs for 18-20 minutes, or until they're cooked through and no longer pink in the center.

5. While the meatballs are baking, heat the olive oil in a large skillet over medium heat. Add the spiralized zucchini "zoodles" and sauté for 3-5 minutes, until they're tender-crisp.

6. Remove the meatballs from the oven and add them to the skillet with the zoodles. Pour the no-sugar-added marinara sauce over the top and toss everything together gently to combine.

7. Serve the turkey meatballs and zoodles immediately, while hot.

This turkey meatball and zoodle dish is a great option for men with diabetes. The turkey is a lean protein, and the zucchini "zoodles" are a low-carb, fiber-rich vegetable. The no-sugar-added marinara sauce adds flavor without adding too many carbs or calories. Enjoy this delicious and diabetes-friendly meal!

45. Pork Tenderloin with Green Beans

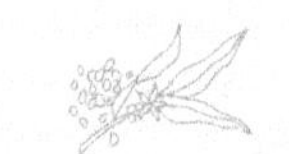

PREP TIME
20 MINUTES

COOK TIME
30 MINUTES

INGREDIENTS:

- 1 lb pork tenderloin, trimmed of any visible fat
- 1 tbsp olive oil
- 1 tsp garlic powder
- 1 tsp dried thyme
- 1/2 tsp salt
- 1/4 tsp black pepper
- 1 lb fresh green beans, trimmed
- 2 tbsp low-sodium soy sauce
- 1 tbsp rice vinegar
- 1 tsp honey
- 1 tsp sesame oil
- 2 cloves garlic, minced
- 1 tsp grated fresh ginger

PROCEDURE:

1. Preheat your oven to 400°F (200°C).

2. In a small bowl, combine the garlic powder, dried thyme, salt, and black pepper. Rub this seasoning mixture all over the pork tenderloin.

3. Heat the olive oil in a large oven-safe skillet over medium-high heat. Sear the pork tenderloin on all sides until it's browned, about 2-3 minutes per side.

4. Transfer the skillet to the preheated oven and roast the pork for 15-20 minutes, or until it reaches an internal temperature of 145°F (63°C). Let the pork rest for 5 minutes before slicing.

5. While the pork is roasting, prepare the green beans. In a medium saucepan, bring 1 inch of water to a boil. Add the green beans and cook for 5-7 minutes, until tender-crisp. Drain and set aside.

6. In a small bowl, whisk together the soy sauce, rice vinegar, honey, sesame oil, minced garlic, and grated ginger.

7. Add the cooked green beans to the soy sauce mixture and toss to coat.

8. Slice the pork tenderloin and serve it with the soy-glazed green beans.

This pork tenderloin and green beans dish is a great option for men with diabetes. The pork is a lean protein, and the green beans are a low-carb vegetable. The soy-ginger sauce adds flavor without adding too many carbs or calories. Enjoy this delicious and diabetes-friendly meal!

46. Stuffed Bell Peppers with Ground Turkey

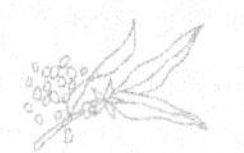
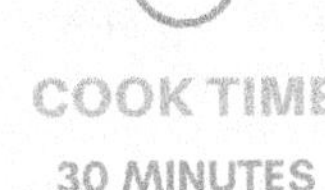

PREP TIME	COOK TIME
20 MINUTES	30 MINUTES

INGREDIENTS:

- 4 large bell peppers (any color), halved lengthwise and seeds removed
- 1 lb ground turkey
- 1 cup cooked brown rice
- 1 (15 oz) can diced tomatoes, no-salt-added
- 1/2 cup diced onion
- 2 cloves garlic, minced
- 1 tsp dried oregano
- 1/2 tsp ground cumin
- 1/4 tsp salt
- 1/4 tsp black pepper
- 1/2 cup shredded low-fat mozzarella cheese

PROCEDURE:

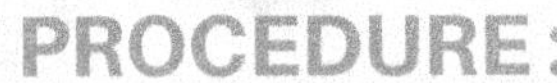

1. Preheat your oven to 375°F (190°C).

2. Place the bell pepper halves in a baking dish and set aside.

3. In a large skillet over medium heat, cook the ground turkey, breaking it up with a wooden spoon, until it's no longer pink, about 5-7 minutes.

4. Add the diced onion and minced garlic to the skillet. Sauté for 2-3 minutes until the onion is translucent.

5. Stir in the cooked brown rice, diced tomatoes, dried oregano, ground cumin, salt, and black pepper. Cook for an additional 2-3 minutes, stirring occasionally.

6. Spoon the turkey and rice mixture into the bell pepper halves, packing it in gently.

7. Top each stuffed pepper half with about 2 tablespoons of shredded mozzarella cheese.

8. Bake the stuffed peppers for 25-30 minutes, or until the peppers are tender and the cheese is melted and bubbly.

9. Serve the stuffed peppers hot.

This stuffed bell pepper dish is a great option for men with diabetes. Ground turkey is a lean protein, and the bell peppers, brown rice, and diced tomatoes provide fiber, vitamins, and minerals. The low-fat mozzarella cheese adds flavor without too many carbs or calories. Enjoy this delicious and diabetes-friendly meal!

47. Grilled Shrimp with Quinoa

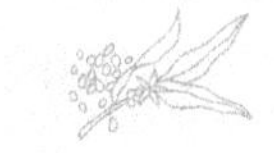

PREP TIME
20 MINUTES

COOK TIME
30 MINUTES

INGREDIENTS:

- 1 lb large shrimp, peeled and deveined
- 2 tbsp olive oil
- 1 tbsp lemon juice
- 1 tsp garlic powder
- 1 tsp dried oregano
- 1/4 tsp salt
- 1/4 tsp black pepper
- 1 cup uncooked quinoa, rinsed
- 2 cups low-sodium chicken or vegetable broth
- 1 cup cherry tomatoes, halved
- 1/4 cup crumbled feta cheese
- 2 tbsp chopped fresh parsley

PROCEDURE:

1. In a large bowl, combine the shrimp, olive oil, lemon juice, garlic powder, dried oregano, salt, and black pepper. Toss to coat the shrimp and let it marinate for 15-20 minutes.

2. Preheat your grill or grill pan to medium-high heat.

3. Thread the marinated shrimp onto skewers (if using wooden skewers, soak them in water for 30 minutes first to prevent burning).

4. Grill the shrimp for 2-3 minutes per side, or until they're opaque and cooked through.

5. While the shrimp is grilling, prepare the quinoa. In a medium saucepan, combine the rinsed quinoa and broth. Bring the mixture to a boil, then reduce the heat, cover, and simmer for 15-20 minutes, or until the quinoa is tender and the liquid is absorbed.

6. Fluff the cooked quinoa with a fork and transfer it to a large bowl. Stir in the halved cherry tomatoes, crumbled feta cheese, and chopped fresh parsley.

7. Serve the grilled shrimp on top of the quinoa salad.

This grilled shrimp and quinoa dish is an excellent choice for men with diabetes. Shrimp is a lean protein, and quinoa is a high-fiber, complex carbohydrate that can help regulate blood sugar levels. The cherry tomatoes, feta cheese, and parsley add flavor and nutrients without too many carbs. Enjoy this delicious and diabetes-friendly meal!

48. Vegetable Stir-Fry with Tofu

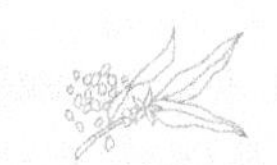

PREP TIME
20 MINUTES

COOK TIME
30 MINUTES

INGREDIENTS:

- 1 block (14 oz) extra-firm tofu, drained and cubed
- 2 tbsp low-sodium soy sauce
- 1 tbsp rice vinegar
- 1 tsp sesame oil
- 1 tbsp olive oil
- 3 cloves garlic, minced
- 1 tbsp grated fresh ginger
- 1 red bell pepper, sliced
- 1 cup broccoli florets
- 1 cup snow peas or snap peas
- 1 cup sliced mushrooms
- 2 green onions, sliced
- 1/4 cup low-sodium vegetable broth
- 1 tsp cornstarch
- Salt and black pepper to taste
- Cooked brown rice (optional)

PROCEDURE:

1. In a medium bowl, combine the cubed tofu, soy sauce, rice vinegar, and sesame oil. Toss to coat the tofu and let it marinate for 15-20 minutes.

2. Heat the olive oil in a large wok or skillet over high heat. Add the marinated tofu and stir-fry for 3-4 minutes, until the tofu is lightly browned.

3. Add the minced garlic and grated ginger to the wok and stir-fry for 1 minute until fragrant.

4. Add the sliced red bell pepper, broccoli florets, snow peas/snap peas, and sliced mushrooms to the wok. Stir-fry for 3-5 minutes, until the vegetables are tender-crisp.

5. In a small bowl, whisk together the vegetable broth and cornstarch. Pour this mixture into the wok and let it simmer for 2-3 minutes, until the sauce has thickened.

6. Stir in the sliced green onions and season the stir-fry with salt and black pepper to taste.

7. Serve the vegetable stir-fry with tofu immediately, either on its own or over a bed of cooked brown rice (if desired).

This vegetable stir-fry with tofu is a great option for men with diabetes. Tofu is a lean, plant-based protein, and the vegetables are low in carbs and high in fiber. The soy sauce, rice vinegar, and cornstarch-thickened broth add flavor without adding too many carbs or calories. Enjoy this delicious and diabetes-friendly meal!

49. Baked Cod with Cauliflower Rice

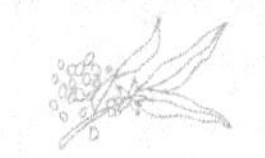

PREP TIME
20 MINUTES

COOK TIME
30 MINUTES

INGREDIENTS:

- 4 (6 oz) cod fillets
- 1 tbsp olive oil
- 1 tsp lemon zest
- 2 tbsp lemon juice
- 1 tsp dried dill
- 1/4 tsp salt
- 1/4 tsp black pepper
- 1 head of cauliflower, riced (about 4 cups riced cauliflower)
- 1 tbsp unsalted butter
- 2 cloves garlic, minced
- 2 tbsp chopped fresh parsley

PROCEDURE:

1. Preheat your oven to 400°F (200°C).

2. Place the cod fillets in a baking dish. In a small bowl, combine the olive oil, lemon zest, lemon juice, dried dill, salt, and black pepper. Brush this mixture over the top of the cod fillets.

3. Bake the cod for 15-18 minutes, or until it flakes easily with a fork and reaches an internal temperature of 145°F (63°C).

4. While the cod is baking, prepare the cauliflower rice. Using a food processor or a box grater, grate the cauliflower florets into rice-sized pieces.

5. In a large skillet, melt the butter over medium heat. Add the riced cauliflower and minced garlic. Sauté for 5-7 minutes, stirring occasionally, until the cauliflower is tender.

6. Remove the cauliflower rice from the heat and stir in the chopped fresh parsley.

7. Serve the baked cod fillets on top of the cauliflower rice.

This baked cod and cauliflower rice dish is an excellent choice for men with diabetes. Cod is a lean, high-protein fish that is also a good source of omega-3 fatty acids. The cauliflower rice is a low-carb, fiber-rich alternative to traditional rice. This meal is both delicious and diabetes-friendly.

50. Chicken Fajitas with Peppers and Onions

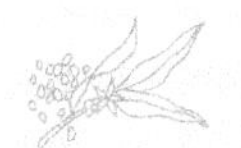 

PREP TIME
20 MINUTES

COOK TIME
30 MINUTES

INGREDIENTS:

- 1 lb boneless, skinless chicken breasts, sliced into thin strips
- 2 tbsp olive oil
- 1 tbsp lime juice
- 1 tsp chili powder
- 1 tsp ground cumin
- 1/2 tsp garlic powder
- 1/4 tsp salt
- 1/4 tsp black pepper
- 1 red bell pepper, sliced
- 1 green bell pepper, sliced
- 1 onion, sliced
- 8 small whole wheat tortillas or lettuce wraps
- Toppings (optional): diced avocado, salsa, low-fat sour cream, shredded cheese

PROCEDURE:

1. In a large bowl, combine the sliced chicken, olive oil, lime juice, chili powder, cumin, garlic powder, salt, and black pepper. Toss to coat the chicken and let it marinate for 15-20 minutes.

2. Heat a large skillet or grill pan over medium-high heat. Add the marinated chicken and cook for 5-7 minutes, stirring occasionally, until the chicken is cooked through and no longer pink.

3. Remove the chicken from the skillet and set it aside. Add the sliced red and green bell peppers and onion to the same skillet. Sauté for 5-7 minutes, until the vegetables are tender-crisp.

4. Return the cooked chicken to the skillet with the peppers and onions. Stir to combine and heat through.

5. Serve the chicken fajita mixture in the whole wheat tortillas or lettuce wraps, allowing guests to customize their fajitas with the desired toppings.

This chicken fajita dish is a great option for men with diabetes. The lean chicken provides protein, while the bell peppers and onions are low-carb, fiber-rich vegetables. The whole wheat tortillas or lettuce wraps offer a healthier alternative to traditional flour tortillas. Customize the fajitas with your choice of diabetes-friendly toppings for a delicious and satisfying meal.

51. Baked Halibut with Mixed Vegetables

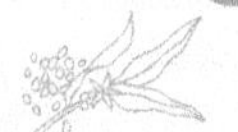

PREP TIME
20 MINUTES

COOK TIME
30 MINUTES

INGREDIENTS :

- 4 (6 oz) halibut fillets
- 1 tbsp olive oil
- 1 tsp lemon zest
- 2 tbsp lemon juice
- 1 tsp dried dill
- 1/4 tsp salt
- 1/4 tsp black pepper
- 1 cup broccoli florets
- 1 cup cauliflower florets
- 1 cup sliced zucchini
- 1 cup sliced yellow squash
- 2 tbsp low-sodium soy sauce
- 1 tsp honey

PROCEDURE :

1. Preheat your oven to 400°F (200°C).

2. Place the halibut fillets in a baking dish. In a small bowl, combine the olive oil, lemon zest, lemon juice, dried dill, salt, and black pepper. Brush this mixture over the top of the halibut fillets.

3. In a large bowl, toss the broccoli florets, cauliflower florets, sliced zucchini, and sliced yellow squash with the soy sauce and honey.

4. Spread the mixed vegetables around the halibut fillets in the baking dish.

5. Bake the halibut and vegetables for 18-22 minutes, or until the fish flakes easily with a fork and the vegetables are tender.

6. Serve the baked halibut immediately, with the roasted mixed vegetables on the side.

This baked halibut and mixed vegetable dish is an excellent choice for men with diabetes. Halibut is a lean, high-protein fish that is also a good source of omega-3 fatty acids. The mixed vegetables provide a variety of nutrients and fiber, while the soy sauce and honey add flavor without too many carbs. This meal is both delicious and diabetes-friendly.

52. Turkey and Vegetable Stuffed Zucchini Boats

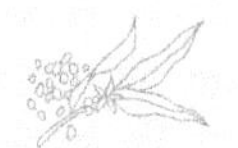

PREP TIME
20 MINUTES

COOK TIME
30 MINUTES

INGREDIENTS :

- 4 medium zucchini, halved lengthwise
- 1 lb ground turkey
- 1 cup diced onion
- 2 cloves garlic, minced
- 1 cup diced bell pepper (any color)
- 1 cup diced mushrooms
- 1 (15 oz) can diced tomatoes, no-salt-added
- 2 tbsp chopped fresh basil
- 1 tsp dried oregano
- 1/4 tsp salt
- 1/4 tsp black pepper
- 1/2 cup shredded low-fat mozzarella cheese

PROCEDURE :

1. Preheat your oven to 375°F (190°C).

2. Scoop out the flesh from the zucchini halves, leaving about 1/4 inch of the zucchini shell. Finely chop the scooped-out zucchini flesh.

3. In a large skillet over medium heat, cook the ground turkey, breaking it up with a wooden spoon, until it's no longer pink, about 5-7 minutes.

4. Add the diced onion, minced garlic, diced bell pepper, and diced mushrooms to the skillet. Sauté for 3-5 minutes until the vegetables are tender.

5. Stir in the chopped zucchini flesh, diced tomatoes, chopped fresh basil, dried oregano, salt, and black pepper. Cook for an additional 2-3 minutes, stirring occasionally.

6. Arrange the zucchini boat halves in a baking dish. Spoon the turkey and vegetable mixture evenly into the zucchini boats.

7. Top each stuffed zucchini boat with about 2 tablespoons of shredded mozzarella cheese.

8. Bake the stuffed zucchini boats for 20-25 minutes, or until the zucchini is tender and the cheese is melted and bubbly. Serve the stuffed zucchini boats hot.

This turkey and vegetable stuffed zucchini boat dish is a great option for men with diabetes. Ground turkey is a lean protein, and the zucchini, bell pepper, and mushrooms provide fiber, vitamins, and minerals. The low-fat mozzarella cheese adds flavor without too many carbs or calories. Enjoy this delicious and diabetes-friendly meal!

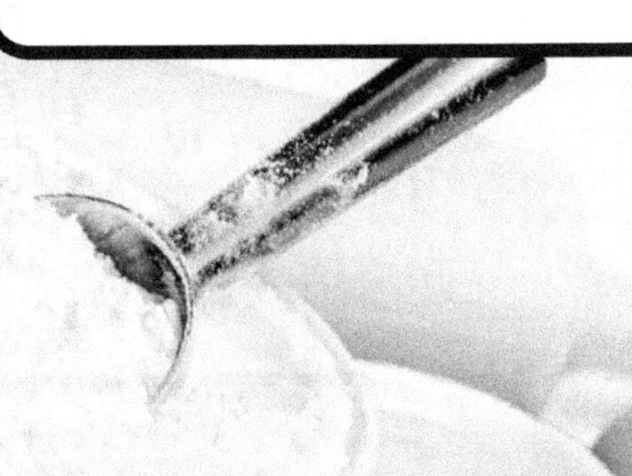

53. Lemon Herb Chicken with Broccoli

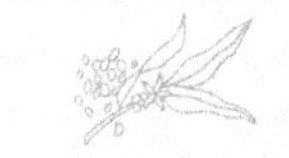 

PREP TIME
20 MINUTES

COOK TIME
30 MINUTES

INGREDIENTS:

- 4 large bell peppers (any color), halved lengthwise and seeds removed
- 1 lb ground turkey
- 1 cup cooked brown rice
- 1 (15 oz) can diced tomatoes, no-salt-added
- 1/2 cup diced onion
- 2 cloves garlic, minced
- 1 tsp dried oregano
- 1/2 tsp ground cumin
- 1/4 tsp salt
- 1/4 tsp black pepper
- 1/2 cup shredded low-fat mozzarella cheese

PROCEDURE:

1. Preheat your oven to 400°F (200°C).

2. In a shallow baking dish, arrange the chicken breasts in a single layer.

3. In a small bowl, combine the olive oil, lemon juice, lemon zest, dried thyme, dried oregano, salt, and black pepper. Whisk to blend.

4. Pour the lemon-herb mixture over the chicken, making sure to coat the chicken evenly.

5. Bake the chicken for 20-25 minutes, or until it reaches an internal temperature of 165°F (74°C).

6. While the chicken is baking, steam the broccoli florets in a steamer basket over boiling water for 5-7 minutes, until tender-crisp.

7. Transfer the steamed broccoli to a bowl and toss with the low-sodium chicken broth.

8. Serve the lemon herb chicken alongside the broccoli.

This lemon herb chicken and broccoli dish is a great option for men with diabetes. The chicken is a lean protein, and the broccoli is a low-carb, fiber-rich vegetable. The lemon and herb seasoning adds flavor without adding too many carbs or calories. This meal is both delicious and diabetes-friendly.

54. Spaghetti Squash with Marinara and Meatballs

PREP TIME
20 MINUTES

COOK TIME
30 MINUTES

INGREDIENTS:

For the Meatballs:
- 1 lb ground turkey
- 1/4 cup whole wheat breadcrumbs
- 1 egg, lightly beaten
- 2 tbsp grated Parmesan cheese
- 2 cloves garlic, minced
- 1 tsp dried oregano
- 1/4 tsp salt
- 1/4 tsp black pepper

For the Spaghetti Squash and Marinara:
- 1 medium spaghetti squash, halved lengthwise and seeds removed
- 1 tbsp olive oil
- 1 (24 oz) jar no-sugar-added marinara sauce
- 2 tbsp fresh basil, chopped (optional)

PROCEDURE:

1. Preheat your oven to 400°F (200°C).

2. Make the meatballs: In a large bowl, combine the ground turkey, breadcrumbs, egg, Parmesan cheese, minced garlic, dried oregano, salt, and black pepper. Mix well until the ingredients are evenly distributed. Roll the mixture into 1-inch meatballs and place them on a baking sheet.

3. Bake the meatballs for 18-20 minutes, or until they're cooked through and no longer pink in the center.

4. While the meatballs are baking, prepare the spaghetti squash. Place the halved squash cut-side down on a baking sheet. Bake for 40-50 minutes, or until the squash is tender and easily shreds with a fork.

5. Remove the spaghetti squash from the oven and use a fork to shred the flesh into spaghetti-like strands.

6. In a large skillet, heat the olive oil over medium heat. Add the shredded spaghetti squash and sauté for 2-3 minutes to heat through.

7. Pour the no-sugar-added marinara sauce over the spaghetti squash and stir to combine.

8. Add the baked turkey meatballs to the skillet and gently toss everything together.

9. Serve the spaghetti squash with marinara and meatballs, garnished with fresh chopped basil if desired.

55. Grilled Pork Chops with Apple Slaw

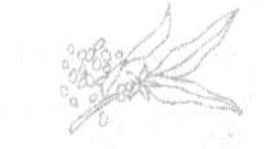 

PREP TIME	COOK TIME
20 MINUTES	30 MINUTES

INGREDIENTS :

For the Pork Chops:
- 4 (6 oz) boneless pork chops
- 1 tbsp olive oil
- 1 tsp garlic powder
- 1 tsp dried thyme
- 1/4 tsp salt
- 1/4 tsp black pepper

For the Apple Slaw:
- 2 cups shredded green cabbage
- 1 cup shredded red cabbage
- 1 medium apple, julienned or grated
- 2 tbsp apple cider vinegar
- 1 tbsp olive oil
- 1 tsp Dijon mustard
- 1 tsp honey
- 1/4 tsp salt
- 1/4 tsp black pepper
- 2 tbsp chopped fresh parsley

PROCEDURE :

1. Preheat your grill or grill pan to medium-high heat.

2. In a small bowl, combine the olive oil, garlic powder, dried thyme, salt, and black pepper. Rub this mixture all over the pork chops.

3. Grill the pork chops for 4-6 minutes per side, or until they reach an internal temperature of 145°F (63°C). Transfer the grilled pork chops to a plate and let them rest for 5 minutes.

4. In a large bowl, combine the shredded green cabbage, shredded red cabbage, and julienned or grated apple.

5. In a small bowl, whisk together the apple cider vinegar, olive oil, Dijon mustard, honey, salt, and black pepper.

6. Pour the dressing over the cabbage and apple mixture and toss to coat.

7. Stir in the chopped fresh parsley.

8. Serve the grilled pork chops with the apple slaw on the side.

This grilled pork chop and apple slaw dish is a great option for men with diabetes. Pork chops are a lean protein, and the cabbage and apple slaw provide fiber, vitamins, and antioxidants. The apple cider vinegar and Dijon mustard dressing adds flavor without too many carbs or calories. Enjoy this delicious and diabetes-friendly meal!

56. Cauliflower Crust Pizza with Veggies

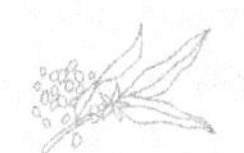

PREP TIME
20 MINUTES

COOK TIME
30 MINUTES

INGREDIENTS:

For the Cauliflower Crust:
- 1 head of cauliflower, riced (about 4 cups riced cauliflower)
- 1 egg, lightly beaten
- 1/4 cup grated Parmesan cheese
- 1/4 tsp salt
- 1/4 tsp black pepper

For the Toppings:
- 1/2 cup no-sugar-added marinara sauce
- 1 cup sliced mushrooms
- 1 cup diced bell peppers (any color)
- 1 cup diced onions
- 1 cup shredded low-fat mozzarella cheese

PROCEDURE:

1. Preheat your oven to 400°F (200°C). Line a baking sheet with parchment paper.

2. To make the cauliflower crust, place the riced cauliflower in a microwave-safe bowl and microwave for 5-7 minutes, until tender. Allow it to cool slightly.

3. Transfer the cooked cauliflower to a clean kitchen towel or cheesecloth and squeeze out as much moisture as possible.

4. In a medium bowl, combine the squeezed cauliflower, beaten egg, Parmesan cheese, salt, and black pepper. Mix well until the ingredients are fully incorporated.

5. Press the cauliflower mixture onto the prepared baking sheet, forming a thin, even crust.

6. Bake the cauliflower crust for 20-25 minutes, or until it's golden brown and crispy.

7. Remove the crust from the oven and top it with the no-sugar-added marinara sauce, sliced mushrooms, diced bell peppers, diced onions, and shredded mozzarella cheese.

8. Return the pizza to the oven and bake for an additional 10-15 minutes, or until the cheese is melted and bubbly. Slice and serve the cauliflower crust pizza hot.

This cauliflower crust pizza is a great option for men with diabetes. The cauliflower crust is low in carbs, and the vegetable toppings provide fiber, vitamins, and minerals. The no-sugar-added marinara sauce and low-fat mozzarella cheese add flavor without too many carbs or calories. Enjoy this delicious and diabetes-friendly pizza!

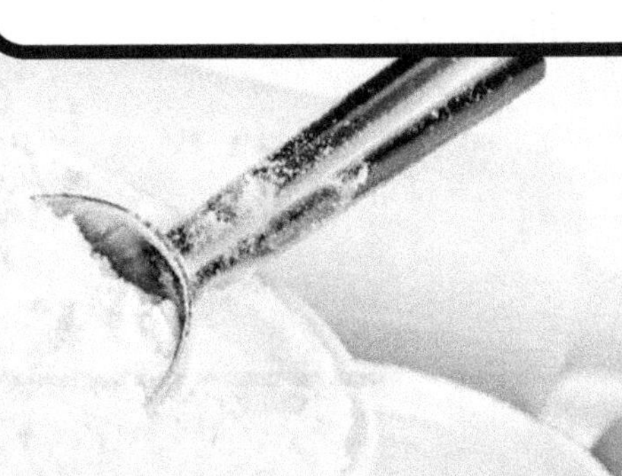

57. Beef and Broccoli Stir-Fry

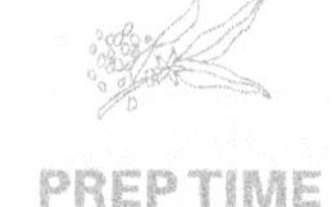

PREP TIME
20 MINUTES

COOK TIME
30 MINUTES

INGREDIENTS:

- 1 lb flank steak, thinly sliced
- 2 tbsp low-sodium soy sauce
- 1 tbsp rice vinegar
- 1 tsp sesame oil
- 1 tbsp olive oil
- 3 cloves garlic, minced
- 1 tbsp grated fresh ginger
- 4 cups broccoli florets
- 1 red bell pepper, sliced
- 1/2 cup low-sodium beef broth
- 1 tsp cornstarch
- Salt and black pepper to taste
- Chopped green onions for garnish (optional)

PROCEDURE:

1. In a medium bowl, combine the sliced flank steak, soy sauce, rice vinegar, and sesame oil. Toss to coat the beef and let it marinate for 15-20 minutes.

2. Heat the olive oil in a large wok or skillet over high heat. Add the marinated beef and stir-fry for 2-3 minutes, until the beef is lightly browned.

3. Add the minced garlic and grated ginger to the wok and stir-fry for 1 minute until fragrant.

4. Add the broccoli florets and sliced red bell pepper to the wok. Stir-fry for 3-5 minutes, until the vegetables are tender-crisp.

5. In a small bowl, whisk together the beef broth and cornstarch. Pour this mixture into the wok and let it simmer for 2-3 minutes, until the sauce has thickened.

6. Season the beef and broccoli stir-fry with salt and black pepper to taste.

7. Serve the stir-fry immediately, garnished with chopped green onions if desired.

This beef and broccoli stir-fry is a great option for men with diabetes. The lean flank steak provides protein, while the broccoli and bell pepper are low-carb, fiber-rich vegetables. The cornstarch-thickened sauce adds flavor without adding too many carbs or calories. Enjoy this delicious and diabetes-friendly meal!

58. Grilled Swordfish with Mango Salsa

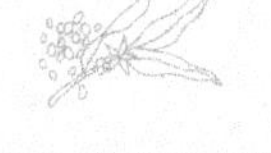 

PREP TIME
20 MINUTES

COOK TIME
30 MINUTES

INGREDIENTS:

For the Mango Salsa:
- 1 ripe mango, diced
- 1/2 red onion, finely chopped
- 1 jalapeño, seeded and finely chopped
- 1/4 cup chopped fresh cilantro
- 2 tbsp fresh lime juice
- 1/4 tsp salt

For the Swordfish:
- 4 (6 oz) swordfish steaks
- 2 tbsp olive oil
- 1 tsp garlic powder
- 1 tsp paprika
- 1/2 tsp salt
- 1/4 tsp black pepper

PROCEDURE:

1. Make the mango salsa: In a medium bowl, combine the diced mango, red onion, jalapeño, cilantro, lime juice, and 1/4 tsp of salt. Stir to mix well and set aside.

2. Prepare the swordfish: Pat the swordfish steaks dry with paper towels. Brush both sides of the steaks with olive oil and season with garlic powder, paprika, salt, and black pepper.

3. Preheat your grill or grill pan to medium-high heat.

4. Grill the swordfish steaks for 3-4 minutes per side, or until they are opaque and flake easily with a fork.

5. Transfer the grilled swordfish steaks to a serving platter and top each one with a generous spoonful of the mango salsa. Serve the grilled swordfish with mango salsa immediately.

Nutritional Information (per serving):
- Calories: 280
- Total Carbs: 12g
- Net Carbs: 10g
- Protein: 35g
- Fat: 12g
- Fiber: 2g

This Grilled Swordfish with Mango Salsa is a delicious and healthy meal option. Swordfish is a lean, high-protein fish that is rich in omega-3 fatty acids. The mango salsa adds a refreshing and flavorful topping, with the sweetness of the mango balancing the heat of the jalapeño. This dish is perfect for a summer grilling night or a light, healthy dinner.

59. Eggplant Parmesan (baked, not fried)

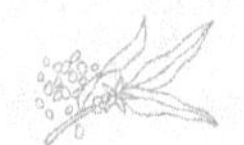

PREP TIME
20 MINUTES

COOK TIME
30 MINUTES

INGREDIENTS :

- 1 large eggplant, sliced into 1/4-inch thick rounds
- 1 cup whole wheat breadcrumbs
- 1/2 cup grated Parmesan cheese
- 1 tsp dried oregano
- 1/2 tsp garlic powder
- 1/4 tsp salt
- 1/4 tsp black pepper
- 1 cup marinara sauce
- 1 cup shredded part-skim mozzarella cheese

PROCEDURE :

1. Preheat your oven to 375°F (190°C). Line a baking sheet with parchment paper.

2. In a shallow bowl, combine the breadcrumbs, Parmesan cheese, oregano, garlic powder, salt, and black pepper.

3. Dip the eggplant slices into the breadcrumb mixture, coating both sides.

4. Arrange the breaded eggplant slices in a single layer on the prepared baking sheet.

5. Bake for 20-25 minutes, flipping the slices halfway through, until the eggplant is tender and the breadcrumbs are golden brown.

6. Remove the baked eggplant slices from the oven and top each one with a spoonful of marinara sauce and a sprinkle of mozzarella cheese.

7. Return the baking sheet to the oven and bake for an additional 5-10 minutes, or until the cheese is melted and bubbly. Serve the Baked Eggplant Parmesan hot.

Nutritional Information (per serving):
- Calories: 180
- Total Carbs: 18g
- Net Carbs: 14g
- Protein: 12g
- Fat: 8g
- Fiber: 4g

This Baked Eggplant Parmesan recipe is a healthier, diabetic-friendly version of the classic dish. By baking the eggplant instead of frying it, you can significantly reduce the amount of fat and calories while still enjoying the delicious flavors.

60. Turkey and Spinach Stuffed Portobello Mushrooms

PREP TIME
20 MINUTES

COOK TIME
30 MINUTES

INGREDIENTS :

- 4 large portobello mushroom caps, stems removed and chopped
- 1 lb ground turkey
- 2 cups fresh spinach, chopped
- 1/2 cup diced onion
- 2 cloves garlic, minced
- 1/4 cup grated Parmesan cheese
- 2 tbsp fresh basil, chopped
- 1 tsp dried oregano
- Salt and pepper to taste

PROCEDURE :

1. Preheat your oven to 375°F (190°C).

2. In a large skillet, cook the ground turkey over medium heat until browned and cooked through, about 5-7 minutes. Drain any excess fat.

3. Add the chopped mushroom stems, onion, and garlic to the skillet. Cook for an additional 3-4 minutes, until the onions are translucent.

4. Stir in the chopped spinach and cook until wilted, about 2 minutes.

5. Remove the skillet from heat and stir in the Parmesan cheese, basil, and oregano. Season with salt and pepper to taste.

6. Arrange the portobello mushroom caps, gill-side up, on a baking sheet. Spoon the turkey and spinach mixture evenly into the mushroom caps.

7. Bake for 15-20 minutes, or until the mushrooms are tender and the filling is hot and bubbly. Serve immediately.

Nutritional Information (per serving):
- Calories: 180
- Total Carbs: 7g
- Net Carbs: 5g
- Protein: 24g
- Fat: 8g
- Fiber: 2g

This recipe is a great option for a diabetic-friendly meal for men as it is low in carbs, high in protein, and provides a good source of fiber and nutrients. The portobello mushrooms are a great low-carb alternative to traditional bread or pasta, and the turkey and spinach filling provides a satisfying and nutritious meal

61. Roasted Brussels Sprouts

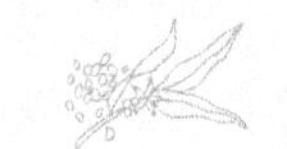 

PREP TIME
20 MINUTES

COOK TIME
30 MINUTES

INGREDIENTS:

- 1 lb Brussels sprouts, trimmed and halved
- 2 tbsp olive oil
- 1 tsp garlic powder
- 1 tsp dried thyme
- 1/4 tsp salt
- 1/4 tsp black pepper

PROCEDURE:

1. Preheat your oven to 400°F (200°C).

2. In a large bowl, toss the trimmed and halved Brussels sprouts with the olive oil, garlic powder, dried thyme, salt, and black pepper until the sprouts are evenly coated.

3. Spread the Brussels sprouts in a single layer on a baking sheet lined with parchment paper.

4. Roast the Brussels sprouts for 20-25 minutes, tossing halfway through, until they are tender and lightly browned.

5. Serve the roasted Brussels sprouts hot.

Nutritional Information (per serving):
- Calories: 80
- Total Carbs: 8g
- Net Carbs: 4g
- Protein: 3g
- Fat: 5g
- Fiber: 4g

This recipe for Roasted Brussels Sprouts is a great option for a diabetic-friendly side dish for men. Brussels sprouts are a low-carb, high-fiber vegetable that can help regulate blood sugar levels. The roasting process brings out the natural sweetness of the sprouts and adds a delicious, crispy texture.

Remember to always consult with your healthcare provider for personalized dietary recommendations based on your individual health needs and goals.

62. Cauliflower Mash

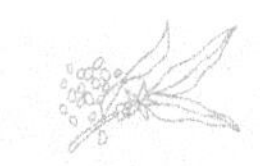

PREP TIME
20 MINUTES

COOK TIME
30 MINUTES

INGREDIENTS:

- 1 head of cauliflower, cut into florets
- 2 tbsp unsalted butter
- 2 tbsp heavy cream (or unsweetened almond milk)
- 1/4 cup grated Parmesan cheese
- 1 tsp garlic powder
- 1/2 tsp salt
- 1/4 tsp black pepper

PROCEDURE:

1. In a large pot, bring a few inches of water to a boil. Add the cauliflower florets, cover, and steam for 10-12 minutes, or until the cauliflower is very tender.

2. Drain the cauliflower and transfer it to a food processor or high-powered blender.

3. Add the butter, heavy cream (or almond milk), Parmesan cheese, garlic powder, salt, and black pepper to the food processor.

4. Blend or process the ingredients until the cauliflower is smooth and creamy, scraping down the sides as needed.

5. Taste and adjust seasoning as desired. Serve the Cauliflower Mash warm.

Nutritional Information (per serving):
- Calories: 100
- Total Carbs: 6g
- Net Carbs: 4g
- Protein: 5g
- Fat: 7g
- Fiber: 2g

This Cauliflower Mash recipe is a great low-carb alternative to traditional mashed potatoes, making it an excellent choice for a diabetic-friendly side dish for men. Cauliflower is a nutrient-dense vegetable that is high in fiber and low in carbs, while the added butter, cream, and Parmesan cheese provide a creamy, satisfying texture and flavor.

This Cauliflower Mash can be enjoyed as a side dish with grilled or roasted meats, fish, or poultry, or even as a base for a low-carb shepherd's pie or other casserole dishes.

63. Sautéed Spinach with Garlic

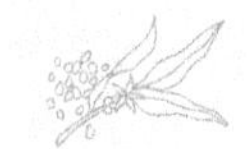 

PREP TIME
20 MINUTES

COOK TIME
30 MINUTES

INGREDIENTS :

- 1 lb fresh spinach, washed and stems removed
- 2 tbsp olive oil
- 3 cloves garlic, minced
- 1/4 tsp salt
- 1/8 tsp black pepper

PROCEDURE :

1. In a large skillet or sauté pan, heat the olive oil over medium heat.

2. Add the minced garlic to the pan and cook for 1-2 minutes, stirring frequently, until fragrant and lightly golden.

3. Add the fresh spinach to the pan in batches, if needed, and sauté for 2-3 minutes, stirring frequently, until the spinach is wilted and tender.

4. Season the sautéed spinach with salt and black pepper, to taste.

5. Serve the Sautéed Spinach with Garlic hot.

Nutritional Information (per serving):
- Calories: 70
- Total Carbs: 4g
- Net Carbs: 2g
- Protein: 3g
- Fat: 5g
- Fiber: 2g

This Sautéed Spinach with Garlic recipe is a great option for a diabetic-friendly side dish for men. Spinach is a nutrient-dense, low-carb vegetable that is high in fiber, vitamins, and minerals. The garlic adds flavor without adding significant carbs or calories.

This dish is easy to prepare and can be a quick and healthy addition to any meal. It pairs well with grilled or roasted meats, fish, or poultry, and can also be enjoyed as a standalone vegetarian dish.

Remember to always consult with your healthcare provider for personalized dietary recommendations based on your individual health needs and goals.

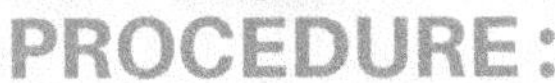
64. Quinoa Pilaf

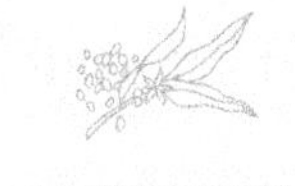

PREP TIME
20 MINUTES

COOK TIME
30 MINUTES

INGREDIENTS :

- 1 cup uncooked quinoa, rinsed
- 2 cups low-sodium chicken or vegetable broth
- 1 tbsp olive oil
- 1 onion, diced
- 2 cloves garlic, minced
- 1 cup diced bell peppers (any color)
- 1 cup diced zucchini
- 1/4 cup chopped fresh parsley
- 1 tsp dried thyme
- 1/4 tsp salt
- 1/4 tsp black pepper

PROCEDURE :

1. In a medium saucepan, combine the rinsed quinoa and broth. Bring the mixture to a boil, then reduce the heat, cover, and simmer for 15-20 minutes, or until the quinoa is tender and the liquid is absorbed.

2. While the quinoa is cooking, heat the olive oil in a large skillet over medium heat. Add the diced onion and sauté for 3-5 minutes until translucent.

3. Add the minced garlic, diced bell peppers, and diced zucchini to the skillet. Sauté for an additional 5-7 minutes, until the vegetables are tender-crisp.

4. Fluff the cooked quinoa with a fork and transfer it to the skillet with the sautéed vegetables. Stir in the chopped fresh parsley, dried thyme, salt, and black pepper.

5. Cook the quinoa pilaf for 2-3 minutes, stirring to combine the ingredients and heat through.

6. Serve the quinoa pilaf warm.

This quinoa pilaf is a great option for men with diabetes. Quinoa is a high-fiber, complex carbohydrate that can help regulate blood sugar levels. The vegetables provide additional fiber, vitamins, and minerals. This dish is a balanced and diabetes-friendly meal that can be enjoyed on its own or as a side dish.

65. Green Bean Almondine

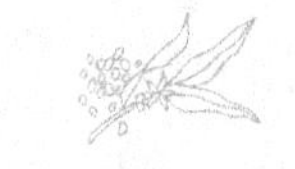

PREP TIME
20 MINUTES

COOK TIME
30 MINUTES

INGREDIENTS:

- 1 lb fresh green beans, trimmed
- 2 tbsp unsalted butter
- 1/4 cup sliced almonds
- 2 cloves garlic, minced
- 1 tbsp lemon juice
- 1/4 tsp salt
- 1/8 tsp black pepper

PROCEDURE:

1. Bring a large pot of salted water to a boil. Add the trimmed green beans and cook for 5-7 minutes, until tender-crisp. Drain the beans and set aside.

2. In a large skillet, melt the butter over medium heat. Add the sliced almonds and cook, stirring frequently, for 2-3 minutes until the almonds are lightly toasted.

3. Add the minced garlic to the skillet and cook for an additional 1 minute, until fragrant.

4. Add the cooked green beans to the skillet and toss to coat with the butter, almonds, and garlic. Cook for 2-3 minutes, until the beans are heated through.

5. Remove the skillet from heat and stir in the lemon juice, salt, and black pepper. Serve the Green Bean Almondine warm.

Nutritional Information (per serving):
- Calories: 110
- Total Carbs: 8g
- Net Carbs: 6g
- Protein: 3g
- Fat: 8g
- Fiber: 2g

This Green Bean Almondine recipe is a classic side dish that features tender-crisp green beans, toasted almonds, and a simple lemon-butter sauce. The combination of flavors and textures makes this a delicious and versatile accompaniment to a variety of main dishes.

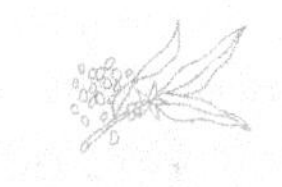

66. Cucumber and Tomato Salad

PREP TIME
20 MINUTES

COOK TIME
30 MINUTES

INGREDIENTS:

- 2 medium cucumbers, sliced
- 2 cups cherry tomatoes, halved
- 1/2 red onion, thinly sliced
- 2 tbsp fresh chopped parsley
- 2 tbsp red wine vinegar
- 1 tbsp olive oil
- 1 tsp Dijon mustard
- 1/4 tsp salt
- 1/8 tsp black pepper

PROCEDURE:

1. In a large bowl, combine the sliced cucumbers, halved cherry tomatoes, and thinly sliced red onion.

2. In a small bowl, whisk together the red wine vinegar, olive oil, Dijon mustard, salt, and black pepper to make the dressing.

3. Pour the dressing over the cucumber, tomato, and onion mixture and toss gently to coat.

4. Sprinkle the fresh chopped parsley over the salad and toss again to combine.

5. Serve the Cucumber and Tomato Salad chilled or at room temperature.

Nutritional Information (per serving):
- Calories: 70
- Total Carbs: 7g
- Net Carbs: 5g
- Protein: 1g
- Fat: 4g
- Fiber: 2g

This Cucumber and Tomato Salad is a refreshing and diabetic-friendly side dish for men. The combination of crisp cucumbers, juicy tomatoes, and tangy red wine vinegar dressing provides a flavorful and low-carb option.

The salad is high in fiber, vitamins, and antioxidants, making it a nutritious addition to any meal. It can be served as a side dish with grilled or roasted meats, fish, or poultry, or enjoyed on its own as a light and healthy snack.

Remember to always consult with your healthcare provider for personalized dietary recommendations based on your individual health needs and goals.

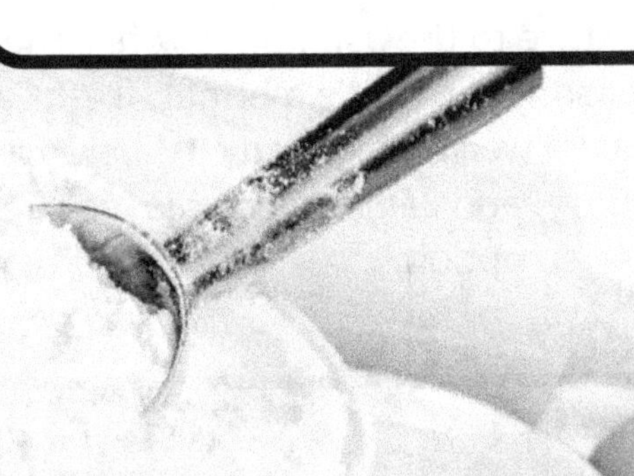

67. Grilled Asparagus

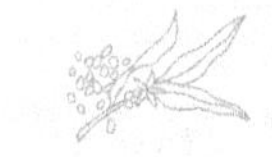 

PREP TIME
20 MINUTES

COOK TIME
30 MINUTES

INGREDIENTS:

- 1 lb fresh asparagus, woody ends trimmed
- 2 tbsp olive oil
- 1 tsp lemon zest
- 1/2 tsp salt
- 1/4 tsp black pepper

PROCEDURE:

1. Preheat your grill or grill pan to medium-high heat.

2. In a large bowl, toss the trimmed asparagus spears with the olive oil, lemon zest, salt, and black pepper until the asparagus is evenly coated.

3. Arrange the seasoned asparagus spears in a single layer on the preheated grill or grill pan.

4. Grill the asparagus for 5-7 minutes, turning occasionally, until it is tender-crisp and lightly charred.

5. Transfer the grilled asparagus to a serving platter or plate. Serve the Grilled Asparagus warm or at room temperature.

Nutritional Information (per serving):
- Calories: 60
- Total Carbs: 4g
- Net Carbs: 3g
- Protein: 3g
- Fat: 4g
- Fiber: 1g

This Grilled Asparagus recipe is a simple and delicious way to enjoy this nutrient-dense vegetable. Asparagus is low in carbs, high in fiber, and a good source of vitamins, minerals, and antioxidants, making it a great choice for a diabetic-friendly side dish.

The grilling process adds a lovely smoky flavor and slightly charred texture to the asparagus, while the lemon zest and seasoning provide a bright, fresh accent. This dish pairs well with grilled or roasted meats, fish, or poultry, and can also be enjoyed as a standalone vegetarian option.

68. Sweet Potato Wedges

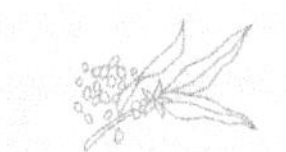

PREP TIME
20 MINUTES

COOK TIME
30 MINUTES

INGREDIENTS :

- 2 medium sweet potatoes, washed and cut into 1/2-inch thick wedges
- 1 tbsp olive oil
- 1 tsp paprika
- 1/2 tsp garlic powder
- 1/4 tsp salt
- 1/4 tsp black pepper

PROCEDURE :

1. Preheat your oven to 400°F (200°C). Line a baking sheet with parchment paper.

2. In a large bowl, toss the sweet potato wedges with the olive oil, paprika, garlic powder, salt, and black pepper until the wedges are evenly coated.

3. Arrange the seasoned sweet potato wedges in a single layer on the prepared baking sheet.

4. Bake for 20-25 minutes, flipping the wedges halfway through, until they are tender and lightly browned.

5. Serve the Sweet Potato Wedges hot.

Nutritional Information (per serving):
- Calories: 100
- Total Carbs: 15g
- Net Carbs: 12g
- Protein: 2g
- Fat: 4g
- Fiber: 3g

This recipe for Sweet Potato Wedges is a great option for a diabetic-friendly side dish for men. Sweet potatoes are a nutrient-dense, complex carbohydrate that can help regulate blood sugar levels. The baking method, rather than frying, helps to keep the carb and calorie counts in check.

The seasoning blend of paprika, garlic powder, salt, and pepper adds flavor without the need for additional sugars or sauces. These Sweet Potato Wedges can be enjoyed as a side dish with grilled or roasted meats, fish, or poultry, or even as a healthy snack on their own

69. Broccoli and Cheese Bake

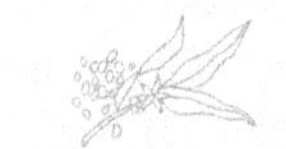 

PREP TIME
20 MINUTES

COOK TIME
30 MINUTES

INGREDIENTS:

- 1 lb broccoli florets
- 1/2 cup shredded cheddar cheese
- 1/4 cup grated Parmesan cheese
- 2 tbsp unsalted butter, melted
- 2 tbsp heavy cream (or unsweetened almond milk)
- 1 clove garlic, minced
- 1/4 tsp salt
- 1/8 tsp black pepper

PROCEDURE:

1. Preheat your oven to 375°F (190°C). Grease a 9x13-inch baking dish.

2. In a large pot, bring a few inches of water to a boil. Add the broccoli florets and cook for 3-5 minutes, until tender-crisp. Drain the broccoli and transfer it to the prepared baking dish.

3. In a small bowl, combine the shredded cheddar cheese, grated Parmesan cheese, melted butter, heavy cream (or almond milk), minced garlic, salt, and black pepper. Stir until well mixed.

4. Pour the cheese mixture over the broccoli in the baking dish and use a spoon to gently toss and coat the broccoli.

5. Bake for 15-20 minutes, or until the cheese is melted and bubbly. Serve the Broccoli and Cheese Bake hot.

Nutritional Information (per serving):
- Calories: 120
- Total Carbs: 6g
- Net Carbs: 4g
- Protein: 7g
- Fat: 9g
- Fiber: 2g

This Broccoli and Cheese Bake is a delicious and diabetic-friendly side dish for men. Broccoli is a low-carb, high-fiber vegetable that is packed with nutrients, while the cheese provides a creamy, satisfying texture and a boost of protein.

The use of heavy cream (or unsweetened almond milk) and a moderate amount of cheese helps to keep the carb and calorie counts in check, making this a great option for those following a diabetic diet.

70. Zucchini Noodles with Pesto

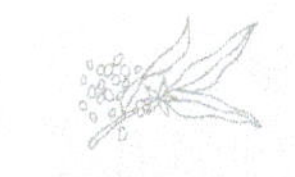

PREP TIME
20 MINUTES

COOK TIME
30 MINUTES

INGREDIENTS:

- 4 medium zucchinis, spiralized or julienned into noodles
- 1/2 cup basil pesto (homemade or store-bought)
- 2 tbsp grated Parmesan cheese
- 1/4 cup cherry tomatoes, halved
- Salt and pepper to taste

PROCEDURE:

1. In a large bowl, combine the zucchini noodles, pesto, and Parmesan cheese. Toss gently to coat the noodles evenly.

2. Add the cherry tomatoes and season with salt and pepper to taste.

3. Serve immediately, or refrigerate until ready to serve.

Nutritional Information (per serving):
- Calories: 120
- Total Carbs: 8g
- Net Carbs: 6g
- Protein: 5g
- Fat: 8g
- Fiber: 2g

This recipe is a great option for a diabetic-friendly meal for men as it is low in carbs, high in fiber, and provides a good source of healthy fats and protein. The zucchini noodles are a great substitute for traditional pasta, and the pesto adds flavor without adding too many carbs. The cherry tomatoes provide a pop of color and additional nutrients.

Remember to always consult with your healthcare provider for personalized dietary recommendations based on your individual health needs and goals.

71. Chia Seed Pudding with Berries

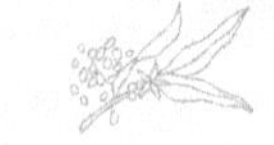

PREP TIME	COOK TIME
20 MINUTES	30 MINUTES

INGREDIENTS :

- 1/4 cup chia seeds
- 1 cup unsweetened almond milk
- 1 tablespoon honey or maple syrup (optional)
- 1/2 cup mixed berries (such as raspberries, blueberries, strawberries)

PROCEDURE :

1. In a medium bowl, whisk together the chia seeds and almond milk until well combined.

2. Cover and refrigerate for at least 2 hours, or overnight, stirring occasionally, until thickened.

3. If desired, stir in the honey or maple syrup to sweeten the pudding.

4. Top the chia seed pudding with the mixed berries just before serving.

Nutritional Information (per serving):
- Calories: 180
- Total Carbs: 16g
- Fiber: 8g
- Net Carbs: 8g
- Protein: 5g
- Fat: 9g

This chia seed pudding is a great option for men with diabetes as it is high in fiber, moderate in carbs, and contains healthy fats from the chia seeds and almond milk. The berries provide antioxidants and additional fiber. The honey or maple syrup is optional, as the berries provide natural sweetness.

Chia seeds are a great source of omega-3 fatty acids, which can help reduce inflammation and improve heart health. This recipe is easy to make and can be prepared in advance for a quick and nutritious breakfast or snack.

72. Greek Yogurt with Nuts and Honey

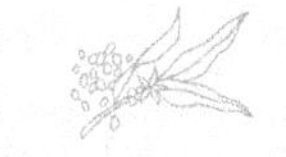 

PREP TIME
20 MINUTES

COOK TIME
30 MINUTES

INGREDIENTS:

- 1 cup plain Greek yogurt (full-fat or low-fat)
- 2 tablespoons chopped walnuts or almonds
- 1 tablespoon raw honey

PROCEDURE:

1. In a small bowl, combine the Greek yogurt, chopped nuts, and honey. Stir gently to combine.

Nutritional Information (per serving):
- Calories: 180
- Total Carbs: 12g
- Fiber: 2g
- Net Carbs: 10g
- Protein: 12g
- Fat: 10g

This recipe is a great option for men with diabetes as it is high in protein, moderate in carbs, and contains healthy fats from the nuts. The Greek yogurt provides probiotics, while the nuts add fiber, vitamins, and minerals. The honey provides a touch of sweetness without spiking blood sugar too much.

Be sure to choose plain, unsweetened Greek yogurt and raw, unprocessed honey for the best nutritional profile. You can also experiment with different nuts like pecans, pistachios, or cashews. Enjoy this as a healthy snack or light breakfast.

73. Apple Crisp with Oats

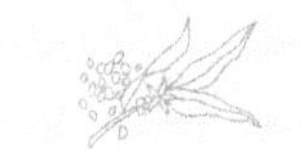

PREP TIME
20 MINUTES

COOK TIME
30 MINUTES

INGREDIENTS:

- 6 cups peeled, cored and sliced apples (about 6-8 medium apples)
- 1 cup old-fashioned oats
- 3/4 cup all-purpose flour
- 3/4 cup brown sugar
- 1/2 cup unsalted butter, softened
- 1 teaspoon ground cinnamon
- 1/4 teaspoon ground nutmeg
- 1/4 teaspoon salt

PROCEDURE:

1. Preheat oven to 350°F. Grease an 8x8 inch baking dish.

2. In a large bowl, toss the sliced apples with 1/4 cup of the brown sugar and the cinnamon. Spread the apples evenly in the prepared baking dish.

3. In a medium bowl, combine the oats, flour, remaining 1/2 cup brown sugar, butter, nutmeg and salt. Use a fork or your fingers to mix until the mixture is crumbly.

4. Sprinkle the oat topping evenly over the apples.

5. Bake for 30-35 minutes, until the apples are tender and the topping is golden brown.

6. Allow to cool for 10-15 minutes before serving. Serve warm, with vanilla ice cream or whipped cream if desired.

Enjoy your homemade apple crisp with the delicious oat topping!

74. Sugar-Free Jello with Whipped Cream

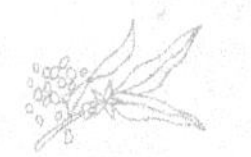 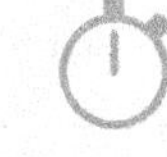

PREP TIME
20 MINUTES

COOK TIME
30 MINUTES

INGREDIENTS:

- 1 (3 oz) package sugar-free Jello (any flavor)
- 2 cups boiling water
- 1 cup cold water
- 1 cup heavy whipping cream
- 1 tsp vanilla extract
- 1-2 tbsp granulated zero-calorie sweetener (like Stevia or Swerve)

PROCEDURE:

1. In a medium bowl, dissolve the sugar-free Jello in the 2 cups of boiling water. Stir until completely dissolved.

2. Add the 1 cup of cold water and stir to combine. Refrigerate the Jello mixture for 1-2 hours, until partially set.

3. In a separate bowl, use a hand mixer to whip the heavy cream until soft peaks form. Add the vanilla and zero-calorie sweetener and continue whipping until stiff peaks form.

4. Fold the whipped cream into the partially set Jello until well combined.

5. Pour the Jello-whipped cream mixture into individual serving dishes or one larger serving bowl.

6. Refrigerate for at least 2 more hours, until fully set.

Serve chilled. This makes a light, creamy, and sugar-free dessert that's perfect for diabetic men. The combination of the sugar-free Jello and sweetened whipped cream provides a delicious treat without the added sugar.

75. Dark Chocolate Avocado Mousse

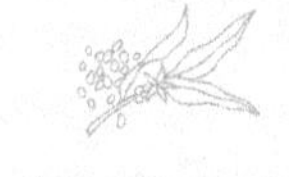

PREP TIME
20 MINUTES

COOK TIME
30 MINUTES

INGREDIENTS :

- 2 ripe avocados, pitted and flesh scooped out
- 1/2 cup unsweetened cocoa powder
- 1/4 cup zero-calorie sweetener (like Stevia or Swerve)
- 1/4 cup unsweetened almond milk
- 1 tsp vanilla extract
- 1/4 tsp sea salt

PROCEDURE :

1. In a food processor or high-powered blender, combine the avocado flesh, cocoa powder, zero-calorie sweetener, almond milk, vanilla, and salt. Blend until completely smooth and creamy, scraping down the sides as needed.

2. Taste and adjust sweetener if desired. The mousse should have a rich, chocolatey flavor.

3. Divide the mousse evenly between 4-6 small serving dishes or ramekins.

4. Cover and refrigerate for at least 2 hours, until chilled and set.

5. Serve chilled, garnished with a sprinkle of cocoa powder, chopped nuts, or fresh berries if desired.

This dark chocolate avocado mousse is a great diabetic-friendly dessert option for men. The avocado provides healthy fats and creaminess, while the cocoa powder and zero-calorie sweetener give it a rich chocolate flavor without the added sugar. It's a satisfying and nutritious treat.

76. Baked Pears with Cinnamon

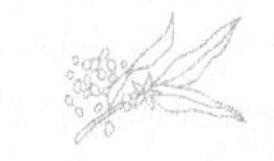 

PREP TIME
20 MINUTES

COOK TIME
30 MINUTES

INGREDIENTS :

- 4 ripe but firm pears, halved and cored
- 2 tbsp unsalted butter, melted
- 2 tbsp ground cinnamon
- 1 tbsp granulated erythritol or other zero-calorie sweetener

PROCEDURE :

1. Preheat your oven to 375°F (190°C). Line a baking sheet with parchment paper.

2. Arrange the pear halves, cut-side up, on the prepared baking sheet.

3. In a small bowl, combine the melted butter, cinnamon, and erythritol (or other sweetener). Stir until well mixed.

4. Spoon the cinnamon-butter mixture evenly over the top of the pear halves, making sure to coat them completely.

5. Bake for 20-25 minutes, or until the pears are tender and the topping is lightly browned. Serve the Baked Pears with Cinnamon warm.

Nutritional Information (per serving):
- Calories: 120
- Total Carbs: 18g
- Net Carbs: 14g
- Protein: 1g
- Fat: 5g
- Fiber: 4g

This Baked Pears with Cinnamon recipe is a delicious and diabetic-friendly dessert or snack option for men. Pears are a naturally sweet fruit that are lower in carbs compared to many other fruits, and the addition of cinnamon and a small amount of zero-calorie sweetener helps to satisfy a sweet craving without spiking blood sugar levels.

The baking process caramelizes the natural sugars in the pears, creating a warm, comforting, and satisfying dessert. This dish can be enjoyed on its own or paired with a small serving of unsweetened Greek yogurt or a sprinkle of chopped nuts for added protein and healthy fats.

77. Berry Parfait with Almonds

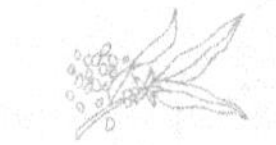

PREP TIME
20 MINUTES

COOK TIME
30 MINUTES

INGREDIENTS :

- 1 cup plain Greek yogurt
- 1/4 cup unsweetened almond milk
- 1 tbsp zero-calorie sweetener (like Stevia or Swerve)
- 1 tsp vanilla extract
- 1 cup mixed berries (such as raspberries, blackberries, blueberries)
- 2 tbsp sliced almonds

PROCEDURE :

1. In a medium bowl, whisk together the Greek yogurt, almond milk, sweetener, and vanilla until well combined.

2. In 2-3 small glasses or parfait dishes, layer the yogurt mixture and the mixed berries, starting and ending with the yogurt.

3. Top each parfait with a sprinkle of sliced almonds.

4. Refrigerate for at least 30 minutes before serving to allow the flavors to meld.

This berry parfait is a great diabetic-friendly dessert option for men. The Greek yogurt provides protein and probiotics, while the berries are full of antioxidants and fiber. The almonds add a nice crunch and healthy fats. The sweetener keeps the sugar content low, making this a satisfying and nutritious treat.

You can adjust the amounts of each ingredient to suit your taste preferences or the number of servings you need. This is a simple, yet delicious and healthy parfait that's perfect for diabetic men.

78. Low-Carb Pumpkin Pie

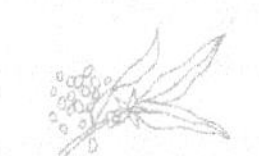

PREP TIME
20 MINUTES

COOK TIME
30 MINUTES

INGREDIENTS:

- 1 1/2 cups almond flour
- 3 tbsp unsalted butter, melted
- 1 tbsp granulated erythritol or other zero-calorie sweetener

Filling
- 1 (15 oz) can pumpkin puree
- 3 large eggs
- 1 cup unsweetened almond milk
- 1/2 cup granulated erythritol or other zero-calorie sweetener
- 1 tsp ground cinnamon
- 1/2 tsp ground ginger
- 1/4 tsp ground nutmeg
- 1/4 tsp ground cloves
- 1/4 tsp salt

PROCEDURE:

For the Crust:
1. Preheat your oven to 350°F (175°C). Grease a 9-inch pie dish.
2. In a medium bowl, mix the almond flour, melted butter, and erythritol until well combined.
3. Press the mixture evenly into the bottom and up the sides of the prepared pie dish.
4. Bake the crust for 10-12 minutes, or until lightly golden. Allow it to cool completely.

For the Filling:
1. In a large bowl, whisk together the pumpkin puree, eggs, almond milk, erythritol, cinnamon, ginger, nutmeg, cloves, and salt until well combined.
2. Pour the pumpkin filling into the prepared crust.
3. Bake the pie for 40-45 minutes, or until the center is almost set.
4. Allow the pie to cool completely before slicing and serving.

This Low-Carb Pumpkin Pie is a delicious and diabetic-friendly dessert option for men. The almond flour crust and the use of zero-calorie sweetener in the filling help to keep the carb and sugar content low, while still providing a rich, creamy pumpkin pie flavor.

Pumpkin is a nutrient-dense ingredient that is low in carbs and high in fiber, vitamins, and antioxidants, making it a great choice for those following a diabetic diet. The addition of spices like cinnamon, ginger, and nutmeg adds warmth and depth of flavor to the pie.

This Low-Carb Pumpkin Pie can be enjoyed as a special treat or dessert, and it's a great option for holiday gatherings or celebrations.

79. Chocolate Chia Pudding

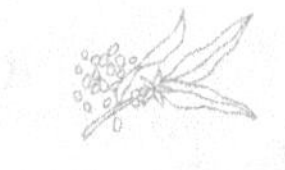 

PREP TIME
20 MINUTES

COOK TIME
30 MINUTES

INGREDIENTS :

- 1/4 cup chia seeds
- 1 1/2 cups unsweetened almond milk
- 2 tbsp unsweetened cocoa powder
- 1-2 tbsp zero-calorie sweetener (like Stevia or Swerve)
- 1 tsp vanilla extract
- Pinch of salt

PROCEDURE :

1. In a medium bowl, whisk together the chia seeds, almond milk, cocoa powder, sweetener, vanilla, and salt until well combined.

2. Cover and refrigerate for at least 2 hours, or up to 5 days, stirring occasionally, until the pudding has thickened.

3. When ready to serve, give the pudding a final stir to incorporate any remaining chia seeds.

4. Divide the chocolate chia pudding evenly between 4 small serving dishes or jars.

5. Top with additional toppings if desired, such as:
   - Fresh berries
   - Chopped nuts or toasted coconut
   - A sprinkle of unsweetened cocoa powder

This chocolate chia pudding is a great diabetic-friendly dessert option for men. The chia seeds provide fiber, protein, and healthy omega-3s, while the cocoa powder and zero-calorie sweetener give it a rich chocolate flavor without the added sugar. The almond milk keeps it dairy-free and low in carbs.

This pudding can be made in advance and stored in the refrigerator for up to 5 days, making it a convenient and nutritious treat. Adjust the sweetener to your desired level of sweetness.

80. Frozen Yogurt Bark with Berries

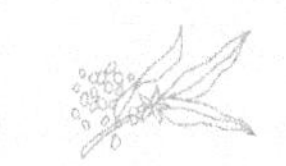

PREP TIME
20 MINUTES

COOK TIME
30 MINUTES

INGREDIENTS:

- 2 cups plain Greek yogurt
- 2 tbsp honey or maple syrup (optional)
- 1 tsp vanilla extract
- 1 cup mixed berries (such as blueberries, raspberries, blackberries)
- 2 tbsp chopped nuts or seeds (such as almonds, walnuts, or pumpkin seeds)

PROCEDURE:

1. Line a baking sheet with parchment paper or a silicone baking mat.

2. In a medium bowl, mix together the Greek yogurt, honey/maple syrup (if using), and vanilla extract until well combined.

3. Spread the yogurt mixture evenly onto the prepared baking sheet, creating a thin, even layer.

4. Sprinkle the mixed berries and chopped nuts/seeds over the top of the yogurt.

5. Place the baking sheet in the freezer and freeze for at least 2-3 hours, or until the yogurt bark is completely frozen.

6. Once frozen, break or cut the yogurt bark into irregular pieces and serve immediately.

7. Store any leftover frozen yogurt bark in an airtight container in the freezer for up to 2 weeks.

This frozen yogurt bark is a refreshing and healthy treat. The Greek yogurt provides protein, while the berries add natural sweetness and antioxidants. The nuts or seeds add a nice crunch and healthy fats. You can adjust the toppings to your liking, such as using different types of berries or adding a drizzle of melted dark chocolate.

This is a great option for a light and satisfying dessert or snack. Enjoy the frozen yogurt bark on its own or paired with a cup of fresh fruit.

81. Green Smoothie with Spinach and Kale

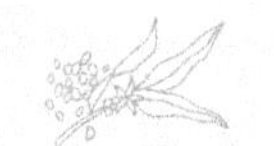

PREP TIME
20 MINUTES

COOK TIME
30 MINUTES

INGREDIENTS:

- 1 cup unsweetened almond milk
- 1 cup packed fresh spinach
- 1 cup packed fresh kale
- 1 medium banana, frozen
- 1/2 cup frozen blueberries
- 1 tbsp ground flaxseed
- 1 tsp honey (optional)

PROCEDURE:

1. In a high-powered blender, combine the unsweetened almond milk, fresh spinach, fresh kale, frozen banana, frozen blueberries, and ground flaxseed.

2. Blend the ingredients on high speed until the smoothie is smooth and creamy, about 1-2 minutes.

3. Taste the smoothie and add the optional honey if you'd like a slightly sweeter flavor. Pour the Green Smoothie into a glass and enjoy immediately.

Nutritional Information (per serving):
- Calories: 200
- Total Carbs: 30g
- Net Carbs: 22g
- Protein: 6g
- Fat: 6g
- Fiber: 8g

This Green Smoothie with Spinach and Kale is a nutrient-dense and diabetic-friendly option for men. The combination of leafy greens, berries, and a small amount of banana provides a good source of fiber, vitamins, and antioxidants, while the almond milk and flaxseed add healthy fats and protein to help keep blood sugar levels stable.

The use of unsweetened almond milk and the optional addition of a small amount of honey help to keep the carb and sugar content in check, making this smoothie a great choice for those following a diabetic diet.

This Green Smoothie can be enjoyed as a healthy breakfast, snack, or even a light meal. It's a great way to incorporate more nutrient-dense greens into your diet

82. Unsweetened Iced Tea

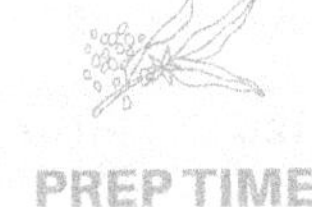

PREP TIME
20 MINUTES

COOK TIME
30 MINUTES

INGREDIENTS:

- 6 black tea bags (or 6 tsp loose leaf black tea)
- 8 cups of water

PROCEDURE:

1. In a large pot, bring the 8 cups of water to a boil.

2. Once the water is boiling, remove it from the heat and add the 6 tea bags (or 6 tsp of loose leaf tea).

3. Allow the tea to steep for 5-7 minutes, depending on your desired strength.

4. Remove the tea bags (or strain out the loose leaf tea) and pour the hot tea into a heat-proof pitcher or container.

5. Allow the tea to cool to room temperature, then refrigerate for at least 2 hours, or until completely chilled.

6. Serve the unsweetened iced tea over ice. You can also add a few lemon slices or mint leaves for extra flavor.

This unsweetened iced tea is a great diabetic-friendly option for men. Black tea is naturally low in calories and carbs, and it provides antioxidants without any added sugars or sweeteners.

The longer you steep the tea, the stronger the flavor will be. You can experiment with different tea varieties, such as green tea or herbal teas, to find your preferred taste.

Unsweetened iced tea is a refreshing and hydrating beverage that's perfect for diabetic men. It's a great alternative to sugary sodas or juices, and it can be enjoyed year-round.

83. Lemon Water

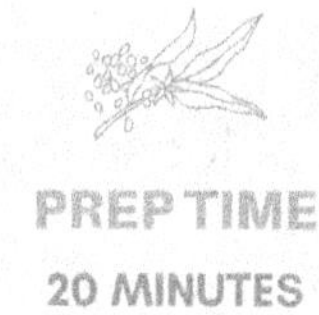

PREP TIME
20 MINUTES

COOK TIME
30 MINUTES

INGREDIENTS:

- 1 lemon, sliced
- 8 cups cold water

PROCEDURE:

1. In a large pitcher or water dispenser, add the sliced lemon.

2. Pour the cold water over the lemon slices and stir gently to combine.

3. Cover the pitcher and refrigerate for at least 2 hours, or up to 8 hours, to allow the lemon flavor to infuse the water.

4. Serve the lemon water chilled, over ice if desired.

5. Refill the pitcher with more water as needed, allowing the lemon to continue infusing.

This lemon water is a great diabetic-friendly option for men. Lemon is a great source of vitamin C and provides a refreshing, tart flavor without any added sugars or sweeteners.

The longer the water infuses, the more intense the lemon flavor will become. You can adjust the amount of lemon slices to suit your taste preferences.

Lemon water is a simple and healthy way to stay hydrated and satisfy your thirst. It's a great alternative to sugary drinks, making it a perfect choice for diabetic men.

You can also try adding a few sprigs of fresh mint or a few slices of cucumber to the lemon water for additional flavor and health benefits.

84. Herbal Tea

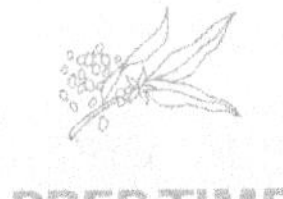

PREP TIME
20 MINUTES

COOK TIME
30 MINUTES

INGREDIENTS :

- 1 tsp dried herbal tea blend (such as chamomile, peppermint, or hibiscus)
- 1 cup boiling water

PROCEDURE :

1. In a mug or teapot, place the 1 tsp of dried herbal tea blend.

2. Pour the boiling water over the tea and let it steep for 5-7 minutes, depending on your desired strength.

3. Strain the tea leaves or remove the tea bag, if using.

4. Serve the herbal tea hot, or allow it to cool and serve it over ice.

5. You can optionally add a slice of lemon or a small amount of zero-calorie sweetener, if desired.

This herbal tea is a great diabetic-friendly option for men. Herbal teas are naturally caffeine-free and low in calories, making them a healthy alternative to sugary drinks.

Some great herbal tea options for diabetic men include:

- Chamomile tea - Soothing and calming
- Peppermint tea - Refreshing and aids digestion
- Hibiscus tea - Tart and high in antioxidants
- Ginger tea - Warming and can help with nausea

You can experiment with different herbal tea blends to find your favorite flavors. The key is to enjoy the tea without any added sugars or sweeteners, which can spike blood sugar levels.

Herbal tea is a comforting and hydrating beverage that's perfect for diabetic men. It's a great way to wind down and support overall health.

85. Cucumber Mint Water

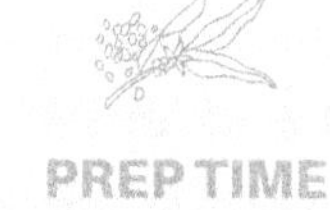 **PREP TIME**
20 MINUTES

 **COOK TIME**
30 MINUTES

INGREDIENTS:

- 1 cucumber, sliced
- 1 cup fresh mint leaves
- 8 cups cold water

PROCEDURE:

1. In a large pitcher or water dispenser, combine the sliced cucumber and fresh mint leaves.

2. Pour the cold water over the cucumber and mint, and stir gently to combine.

3. Cover the pitcher and refrigerate for at least 2 hours, or up to 8 hours, to allow the flavors to infuse the water.

4. Serve the cucumber mint water chilled, over ice if desired.

5. Refill the pitcher with more water as needed, allowing the cucumber and mint to continue infusing.

This cucumber mint water is a great diabetic-friendly option for men. The cucumber provides a refreshing, hydrating element, while the mint adds a bright, herbal flavor without any added sugars or sweeteners.

The longer the water infuses, the more intense the cucumber and mint flavors will become. You can experiment with the ratio of cucumber to mint to find your perfect balance.

This infused water is a great way to stay hydrated and satisfy your thirst while avoiding sugary drinks. It's a healthy and delicious alternative that's perfect for diabetic men.

86. Coconut Water

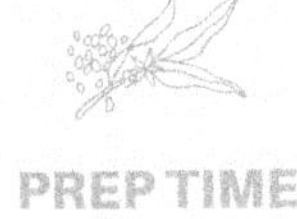

PREP TIME
20 MINUTES

COOK TIME
30 MINUTES

INGREDIENTS:

- 1 cup coconut water
- 1 cup frozen pineapple chunks
- 1 banana, frozen
- 1 cup spinach or kale
- 1 tbsp chia seeds (optional)
- 1 tbsp honey or maple syrup (optional)

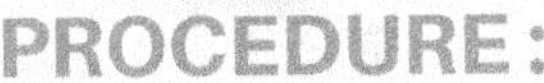

PROCEDURE:

1. Add all the ingredients to a high-powered blender.

2. Blend on high speed until smooth and creamy, about 1-2 minutes.

3. Taste and adjust sweetness if needed, adding a bit more honey or maple syrup.

4. Pour into a glass and enjoy immediately.

Tips:

- Use ripe, frozen bananas for a thicker, creamier smoothie.

- Add a scoop of protein powder for extra nutrition.

- Top with shredded coconut, sliced almonds, or a drizzle of nut butter.

- Substitute the fruit with other frozen options like mango, berries, or peaches.

- For a thinner consistency, add more coconut water.

The coconut water provides natural electrolytes and hydration, while the fruit and greens pack in vitamins, minerals, and fiber. This smoothie makes a refreshing and nutritious breakfast or snack.

87. Almond Milk Smoothie

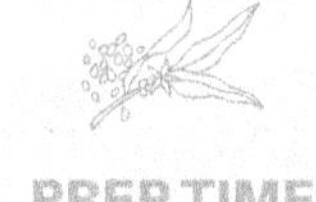 

PREP TIME
20 MINUTES

COOK TIME
30 MINUTES

INGREDIENTS:

- 1 cup unsweetened almond milk
- 1/2 cup frozen berries (such as blueberries, raspberries, or strawberries)
- 1/2 banana, frozen
- 1 tbsp almond butter
- 1 tbsp ground flaxseed
- 1 tsp vanilla extract
- 1-2 tsp zero-calorie sweetener (optional)

PROCEDURE:

1. In a high-powered blender, combine the unsweetened almond milk, frozen berries, frozen banana, almond butter, ground flaxseed, and vanilla extract.

2. Blend on high speed until the mixture is smooth and creamy, about 1-2 minutes.

3. Taste the smoothie and add 1-2 tsp of zero-calorie sweetener if desired, depending on the sweetness of the fruit.

4. Pour the smoothie into a glass and enjoy immediately.

This almond milk smoothie is a great diabetic-friendly option for men. The unsweetened almond milk provides a creamy base without any added sugars. The frozen fruit adds natural sweetness and fiber, while the almond butter and flaxseed provide healthy fats and protein to help keep you feeling full and satisfied.

The zero-calorie sweetener is optional, as the fruit should provide enough sweetness. However, you can adjust the amount to your personal taste preferences.

This smoothie is a nutritious and delicious way for diabetic men to enjoy a refreshing and satisfying treat. It's a great option for breakfast, a snack, or even a light dessert.

88. Sugar-Free Lemonade

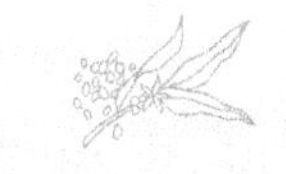

PREP TIME
20 MINUTES

COOK TIME
30 MINUTES

INGREDIENTS:

- 1 cup freshly squeezed lemon juice (about 4-6 lemons)
- 4 cups water
- 1/4 cup zero-calorie sweetener (such as stevia, erythritol, or monk fruit sweetener)
- Ice cubes

PROCEDURE:

1. In a pitcher, combine the lemon juice, water, and sweetener. Stir until the sweetener is fully dissolved.

2. Taste and adjust sweetener amount to your preference. Start with 1/4 cup and add more if you want it sweeter.

3. Fill glasses with ice cubes and pour the lemonade over the ice.

4. Serve immediately and enjoy your refreshing, sugar-free lemonade!

You can also add sliced lemon or mint leaves as a garnish. This recipe is a great low-calorie, diabetic-friendly alternative to regular lemonade. The key is using a zero-calorie sweetener instead of sugar.

89. Berry Infused Water

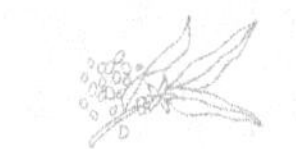

PREP TIME
20 MINUTES

COOK TIME
30 MINUTES

INGREDIENTS:

- 1 cup mixed berries (such as raspberries, blackberries, blueberries)
- 1 lemon, sliced
- 1 lime, sliced
- 8 cups cold water

PROCEDURE:

1. In a large pitcher or water dispenser, combine the mixed berries, lemon slices, and lime slices.

2. Pour the cold water over the fruit and stir gently to combine.

3. Cover the pitcher and refrigerate for at least 2 hours, or up to 8 hours, to allow the flavors to infuse the water.

4. Serve the berry infused water chilled, over ice if desired.

5. Refill the pitcher with more water as needed, allowing the fruit to continue infusing.

This berry infused water is a great diabetic-friendly option for men. The berries provide natural sweetness and antioxidants, while the citrus fruits add a refreshing tartness without any added sugars.

The longer the water infuses, the more intense the fruit flavor will become. You can experiment with different berry and citrus combinations to find your favorite flavor profile.

This infused water is a great way to stay hydrated and satisfy your thirst while avoiding sugary drinks. It's a healthy and delicious alternative that's perfect for diabetic men.

90. Decaf Coffee

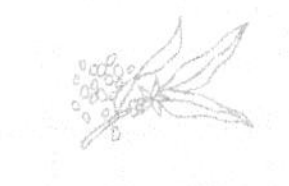

PREP TIME
20 MINUTES

COOK TIME
30 MINUTES

INGREDIENTS :

- 1/2 cup ground decaf coffee beans
- 4 cups cold water

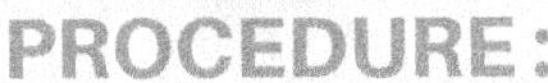

PROCEDURE :

1. In a coffee maker, add the ground decaf coffee beans to the filter.

2. Pour the 4 cups of cold water into the coffee maker's water reservoir.

3. Turn on the coffee maker and brew the decaf coffee.

4. Once brewed, pour the decaf coffee into mugs.

5. You can add any desired toppings or mix-ins, such as milk, cream, sugar, or sweetener.

Tips for making great decaf coffee:

- Use a high-quality decaf coffee bean for the best flavor.

- Adjust the coffee-to-water ratio to your taste preference. Start with 1/2 cup coffee per 4 cups water.

- For a stronger decaf, use more coffee grounds. For a milder decaf, use less.

- Consider using a French press or pour over method for a richer, more flavorful decaf.

- Store decaf coffee beans in an airtight container in a cool, dark place to preserve freshness.

Enjoy your delicious, caffeine-free decaf coffee!

91. Canned Tuna with Avocado

PREP TIME
20 MINUTES

COOK TIME
30 MINUTES

INGREDIENTS :

- 1 (5 oz) can of tuna, drained
- 1 ripe avocado, diced
- 1 tbsp mayonnaise
- 1 tsp lemon juice
- Salt and pepper to taste

PROCEDURE :

1. In a medium bowl, gently mix together the drained tuna, diced avocado, mayonnaise, and lemon juice until well combined.

2. Season with salt and pepper to taste.

3. Serve the tuna and avocado mixture on its own, on top of crackers or toast, or stuffed into halved tomatoes or lettuce leaves.

Tips:
- Use a high-quality canned tuna, preferably packed in water or olive oil.

- Adjust the amount of mayonnaise to your desired creaminess.

- Add a sprinkle of paprika or cayenne pepper for a little kick.

- For extra crunch, mix in some diced celery or red onion.

- Garnish with fresh herbs like parsley or dill.

This tuna and avocado combination makes a nutritious, protein-packed, and delicious snack or light meal. The healthy fats from the avocado pair perfectly with the tuna. Enjoy!

92. Rotisserie Chicken with Mixed Greens

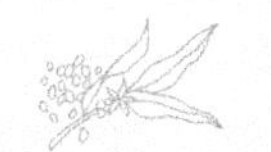 

PREP TIME
20 MINUTES

COOK TIME
30 MINUTES

INGREDIENTS :

- 1 store-bought rotisserie chicken, skin removed and meat shredded or chopped
- 6 cups mixed greens (such as spinach, arugula, kale)
- 1 cup cherry tomatoes, halved
- 1/2 cup sliced cucumber
- 2 tbsp olive oil
- 1 tbsp balsamic vinegar
- 1 tsp Dijon mustard
- Salt and pepper to taste

PROCEDURE :

1. In a large salad bowl, combine the shredded rotisserie chicken, mixed greens, cherry tomatoes, and sliced cucumber.

2. In a small bowl, whisk together the olive oil, balsamic vinegar, and Dijon mustard. Season with salt and pepper.

3. Drizzle the dressing over the salad and toss gently to coat.

4. Serve immediately.

Nutritional Information (per serving):
- Calories: 300
- Total Fat: 16g
- Saturated Fat: 3g
- Carbohydrates: 10g
- Fiber: 4g
- Protein: 32g
- Sodium: 450mg

This rotisserie chicken and mixed greens salad is a great option for men with diabetes. It's high in protein, low in carbs, and provides a variety of nutrient-dense vegetables. The healthy fats from the olive oil and avocado help to keep you feeling full and satisfied. Adjust the portion sizes as needed to fit your individual dietary needs.

93. Veggie and Hummus Wrap

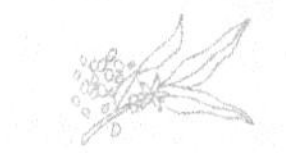

PREP TIME
20 MINUTES

COOK TIME
30 MINUTES

INGREDIENTS:

- 1 (8-inch) whole wheat tortilla or wrap
- 2 tbsp hummus
- 1/2 cup mixed greens (spinach, arugula, etc.)
- 1/4 cup sliced cucumber
- 1/4 cup sliced bell pepper
- 1/4 cup shredded carrots
- 1 tbsp crumbled feta cheese (optional)
- Salt and pepper to taste

PROCEDURE:

1. Spread the hummus evenly over the tortilla or wrap, leaving a 1-inch border.

2. Layer the mixed greens, sliced cucumber, bell pepper, and shredded carrots on top of the hummus.

3. Sprinkle the crumbled feta cheese over the vegetables, if using.

4. Season with salt and pepper to taste.

5. Fold the bottom of the tortilla up, then fold in the sides and roll up tightly to create a wrap.

6. Cut the wrap in half diagonally and serve.

Nutritional Information (per serving):
- Calories: 250
- Total Fat: 10g
- Saturated Fat: 2g
- Carbohydrates: 30g
- Fiber: 7g
- Protein: 10g
- Sodium: 450mg

This veggie and hummus wrap is a great option for men with diabetes. It's high in fiber, low in carbs, and provides a variety of nutrient-dense vegetables. The hummus adds protein and healthy fats to help keep you feeling full and satisfied. Adjust the portion sizes as needed to fit your individual dietary needs.

94. Egg Salad on Whole Grain Bread

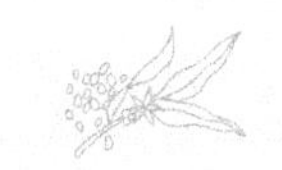

PREP TIME
20 MINUTES

COOK TIME
30 MINUTES

INGREDIENTS :

- 6 hard-boiled eggs, peeled and chopped
- 2 tbsp plain Greek yogurt
- 1 tbsp Dijon mustard
- 1 tbsp chopped fresh dill (or 1 tsp dried dill)
- 2 tbsp finely chopped celery
- 1 tbsp finely chopped red onion
- Salt and pepper to taste
- 4 slices of whole grain bread

PROCEDURE :

1. In a medium bowl, combine the chopped hard-boiled eggs, Greek yogurt, Dijon mustard, dill, celery, and red onion. Mix well until fully incorporated.

2. Season the egg salad with salt and pepper to taste.

3. Toast the whole grain bread slices.

4. Spread the egg salad evenly over two of the toast slices, then top with the remaining two slices of toast to create sandwiches.

Nutritional Information (per serving, 1 sandwich):
- Calories: 250
- Total Fat: 10g
- Saturated Fat: 2g
- Carbohydrates: 25g
- Fiber: 5g
- Protein: 15g
- Sodium: 450mg

This egg salad on whole grain bread is a great option for men with diabetes. The eggs provide a good source of protein, while the whole grain bread offers fiber and complex carbohydrates. The Greek yogurt helps to keep the egg salad creamy without adding too much fat or calories. Adjust the portion sizes as needed to fit your individual dietary needs.

95. Turkey and Cheese Roll-Ups

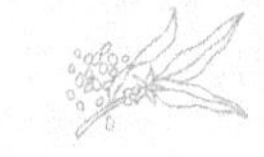 

PREP TIME
20 MINUTES

COOK TIME
30 MINUTES

INGREDIENTS :

- 8 slices of deli-style turkey breast
- 4 slices of low-fat cheddar or Swiss cheese
- 1 tbsp Dijon mustard
- 1 tbsp chopped fresh parsley (optional)

PROCEDURE :

1. Lay the turkey slices out flat on a clean surface.

2. Place a slice of cheese on each turkey slice.

3. Spread a thin layer of Dijon mustard over the cheese.

4. Sprinkle the chopped parsley over the mustard, if using.

5. Carefully roll up each turkey slice, starting from the short end and rolling tightly.

6. Secure the roll-ups with toothpicks or cut them in half diagonally to serve.

Nutritional Information (per serving, 2 roll-ups):
- Calories: 150
- Total Fat: 6g
- Saturated Fat: 3g
- Carbohydrates: 2g
- Fiber: 0g
- Protein: 20g
- Sodium: 650mg

These turkey and cheese roll-ups are a great diabetic-friendly option for men. The lean turkey breast provides a good source of protein, while the low-fat cheese adds a touch of creaminess. The Dijon mustard provides flavor without adding extra calories or carbs. This makes for a quick and easy snack or light meal that is both satisfying and nutritious.

Adjust the portion sizes as needed to fit your individual dietary needs. You can also try using different types of cheese or adding other vegetables, such as sliced cucumber or bell pepper, to the roll-ups.

96. Baked Chicken Tenders

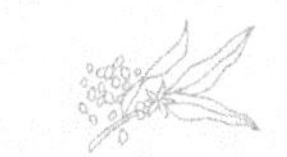 

PREP TIME
20 MINUTES

COOK TIME
30 MINUTES

INGREDIENTS :

- 1 lb boneless, skinless chicken tenders
- 1/2 cup whole wheat breadcrumbs
- 2 tbsp grated Parmesan cheese
- 1 tsp dried oregano
- 1/2 tsp garlic powder
- 1/4 tsp paprika
- Salt and pepper to taste
- 1 tbsp olive oil

PROCEDURE :

1. Preheat the oven to 400°F. Line a baking sheet with parchment paper or a silicone baking mat.

2. In a shallow bowl, combine the breadcrumbs, Parmesan cheese, oregano, garlic powder, paprika, salt, and pepper.

3. Drizzle the olive oil over the chicken tenders and toss to coat.

4. Dredge the chicken tenders in the breadcrumb mixture, pressing gently to help the coating adhere.

5. Arrange the breaded chicken tenders in a single layer on the prepared baking sheet.

6. Bake for 15-18 minutes, flipping halfway through, until the chicken is cooked through and the breading is golden brown. Serve the baked chicken tenders immediately.

Nutritional Information (per serving, 3 chicken tenders):
- Calories: 220
- Total Fat: 8g
- Saturated Fat: 2g
- Carbohydrates: 12g
- Fiber: 2g
- Protein: 25g
- Sodium: 350mg

These baked chicken tenders are a great diabetic-friendly option for men. The whole wheat breadcrumbs and Parmesan cheese provide a crispy coating without the need for frying. The lean protein from the chicken and the minimal added fat make this a healthy and satisfying meal. Adjust the portion sizes as needed to fit your individual dietary needs.

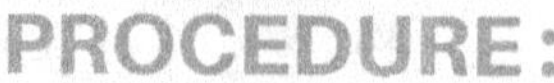
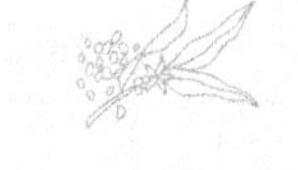

97. Shrimp Cocktail

PROCEDURE:

PREP TIME
20 MINUTES

COOK TIME
30 MINUTES

INGREDIENTS:

- 1 lb cooked, peeled, and deveined shrimp
- 1/2 cup low-sodium cocktail sauce
- 1 tbsp fresh lemon juice
- 1 tbsp chopped fresh parsley
- Salt and pepper to taste

1. In a medium bowl, combine the cooked shrimp, cocktail sauce, lemon juice, and parsley. Toss gently to coat the shrimp.

2. Season with salt and pepper to taste.

3. Cover and refrigerate for at least 30 minutes to allow the flavors to meld.

4. Serve the shrimp cocktail chilled, with lemon wedges on the side.

Nutritional Information (per serving, 5 shrimp with 2 tbsp cocktail sauce):
- Calories: 100
- Total Fat: 1g
- Saturated Fat: 0g
- Carbohydrates: 5g
- Fiber: 0g
- Protein: 15g
- Sodium: 350mg

This shrimp cocktail is a great diabetic-friendly option for men. Shrimp is a lean protein that is low in carbs and calories, making it a great choice for those with diabetes. The cocktail sauce provides a flavorful dipping sauce without adding too many carbs or calories.

To make this even more diabetic-friendly, you can use a low-sugar or no-sugar-added cocktail sauce. You can also serve the shrimp with a side of fresh lemon wedges or a small salad for added nutrients.

Adjust the portion sizes as needed to fit your individual dietary needs. Enjoy this refreshing and healthy shrimp cocktail!

98. Grilled Veggie Skewers

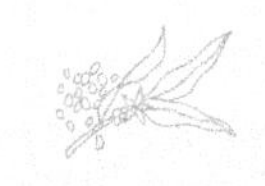

PREP TIME
20 MINUTES

COOK TIME
30 MINUTES

INGREDIENTS:

- 1 zucchini, cut into 1-inch pieces
- 1 yellow squash, cut into 1-inch pieces
- 1 red bell pepper, cut into 1-inch pieces
- 1 red onion, cut into 1-inch pieces
- 8 oz mushrooms, halved
- 2 tbsp olive oil
- 1 tsp dried oregano
- 1 tsp dried basil
- Salt and pepper to taste

PROCEDURE:

1. Preheat grill or grill pan to medium-high heat.
2. In a large bowl, toss the cut vegetables with the olive oil, oregano, basil, salt, and pepper until well coated.
3. Thread the vegetables onto skewers, alternating the different types.
4. Grill the veggie skewers for 12-15 minutes, turning occasionally, until the vegetables are tender and lightly charred.
5. Serve the grilled veggie skewers hot.

Nutritional Information (per serving, 2 skewers):
- Calories: 120
- Total Fat: 7g
- Saturated Fat: 1g
- Carbohydrates: 12g
- Fiber: 3g
- Protein: 3g
- Sodium: 150mg

These grilled veggie skewers are a great diabetic-friendly option for men. They are low in calories, high in fiber, and packed with a variety of nutrient-dense vegetables. The grilling adds a delicious smoky flavor to the veggies. Adjust the portion sizes as needed to fit your individual dietary needs.

You can also try adding other vegetables like cherry tomatoes, eggplant, or asparagus to the skewers. Serve the grilled veggies as a side dish or as part of a larger meal.

99. Baked Salmon Patties

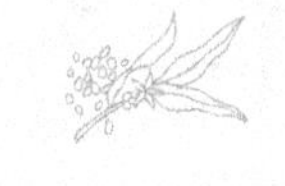

PREP TIME
20 MINUTES

COOK TIME
30 MINUTES

INGREDIENTS:

- 2 (15 oz) cans of salmon, drained and flaked
- 1 egg, lightly beaten
- 1/4 cup whole wheat breadcrumbs
- 2 tbsp chopped fresh parsley
- 1 tbsp Dijon mustard
- 1 tsp lemon juice
- 1/4 tsp garlic powder
- Salt and pepper to taste
- 1 tbsp olive oil

PROCEDURE:

1. Preheat the oven to 400°F. Line a baking sheet with parchment paper.

2. In a medium bowl, combine the flaked salmon, egg, breadcrumbs, parsley, Dijon mustard, lemon juice, garlic powder, salt, and pepper. Mix well until fully incorporated.

3. Divide the salmon mixture into 8 equal portions and shape them into patties, about 1/2 inch thick.

4. Place the salmon patties on the prepared baking sheet. Brush the tops of the patties lightly with the olive oil.

5. Bake for 15-18 minutes, flipping halfway through, until the patties are golden brown and cooked through.

6. Serve the baked salmon patties warm, with lemon wedges on the side.

Nutritional Information (per serving, 2 patties):
- Calories: 200
- Total Fat: 9g
- Saturated Fat: 2g
- Carbohydrates: 6g
- Fiber: 1g
- Protein: 22g
- Sodium: 400mg

These baked salmon patties are a great diabetic-friendly option for men. Salmon is a rich source of heart-healthy omega-3 fatty acids, and the baking method helps to keep the patties low in fat and calories. The whole wheat breadcrumbs provide fiber, while the Dijon mustard and lemon juice add flavor without added sugars.

100. Zucchini Boats with Ground Beef

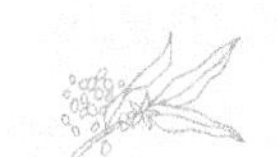

PREP TIME
20 MINUTES

COOK TIME
30 MINUTES

INGREDIENTS:

- 4 medium zucchini, halved lengthwise
- 1 lb lean ground beef
- 1/2 cup diced onion
- 2 cloves garlic, minced
- 1 (15 oz) can diced tomatoes
- 1 tsp dried oregano
- 1/2 tsp dried basil
- 1/4 tsp red pepper flakes (optional)
- 1/2 cup shredded low-fat mozzarella cheese
- Salt and pepper to taste

PROCEDURE:

1. Preheat the oven to 375°F. Spray a baking dish with non-stick cooking spray.

2. Scoop out the flesh from the zucchini halves, leaving about 1/4 inch of the zucchini shell. Chop the scooped-out zucchini flesh.

3. In a large skillet, cook the ground beef over medium heat, breaking it up as it cooks, until no longer pink, about 5-7 minutes. Drain any excess fat.

4. Add the diced onion and chopped zucchini flesh to the skillet. Cook for 3-4 minutes, until the vegetables are tender.

5. Stir in the garlic, diced tomatoes, oregano, basil, and red pepper flakes (if using). Season with salt and pepper to taste.

6. Arrange the zucchini boats in the prepared baking dish. Spoon the ground beef mixture evenly into the zucchini boats.

7. Top the filled zucchini boats with the shredded mozzarella cheese.

8. Bake for 20-25 minutes, or until the zucchini is tender and the cheese is melted and bubbly. Serve hot.

Nutritional Information (per serving, 2 zucchini boat halves):
- Calories: 250
- Total Fat: 12g
- Saturated Fat: 5g
- Carbohydrates: 12g
- Fiber: 3g
- Protein: 25g
- Sodium: 400mg

101. Grilled Chicken with Quinoa and Veggies

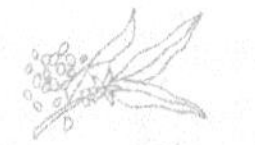

PREP TIME
20 MINUTES

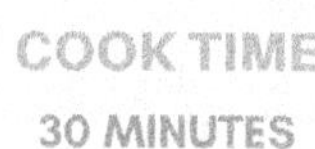

COOK TIME
30 MINUTES

INGREDIENTS :

- 4 boneless, skinless chicken breasts
- 1 cup uncooked quinoa
- 2 cups low-sodium chicken broth
- 1 cup diced zucchini
- 1 cup diced bell pepper
- 1/2 cup diced onion
- 2 cloves garlic, minced
- 2 tbsp olive oil
- 1 tsp dried oregano
- 1 tsp dried basil
- Salt and pepper to taste

PROCEDURE :

1. Preheat grill or grill pan to medium-high heat.

2. Season the chicken breasts with salt, pepper, and any other desired seasonings.

3. Grill the chicken for 5-7 minutes per side, or until cooked through. Set aside and keep warm.

4. In a medium saucepan, combine the quinoa and chicken broth. Bring to a boil, then reduce heat to low, cover, and simmer for 15-20 minutes, or until quinoa is tender and liquid is absorbed.

5. In a large skillet, heat the olive oil over medium heat. Add the diced zucchini, bell pepper, onion, and garlic. Sauté for 5-7 minutes, or until vegetables are tender.

6. Fluff the cooked quinoa with a fork and stir in the sautéed vegetables. Season with oregano, basil, salt, and pepper. Serve the grilled chicken on top of the quinoa and vegetable mixture.

Nutritional Information (per serving, 1 chicken breast with 1 cup quinoa and veggies):
- Calories: 400
- Total Fat: 12g
- Saturated Fat: 2g
- Carbohydrates: 35g
- Fiber: 5g
- Protein: 40g
- Sodium: 350mg

This grilled chicken with quinoa and veggies is a great diabetic-friendly option for men. The lean protein from the chicken, complex carbohydrates from the quinoa, and fiber-rich vegetables make it a well-balanced and nutrient-dense meal. Adjust the portion sizes as needed to fit your individual dietary needs.

102. Salmon with Roasted Vegetables

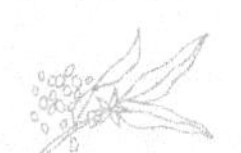

PREP TIME
20 MINUTES

COOK TIME
30 MINUTES

INGREDIENTS:

- 4 (6 oz) salmon fillets
- 2 tbsp olive oil, divided
- 1 tsp dried dill
- Salt and pepper to taste
- 1 cup broccoli florets
- 1 cup sliced zucchini
- 1 cup sliced bell pepper
- 1 cup sliced onion
- 2 cloves garlic, minced
- 1 tbsp lemon juice

PROCEDURE:

1. Preheat the oven to 400°F. Line a large baking sheet with parchment paper.

2. Place the salmon fillets on one side of the baking sheet. Drizzle 1 tbsp of the olive oil over the salmon and sprinkle with the dried dill, salt, and pepper.

3. In a large bowl, toss the broccoli, zucchini, bell pepper, and onion with the remaining 1 tbsp of olive oil, garlic, salt, and pepper. Spread the seasoned vegetables on the other side of the baking sheet, arranging them in a single layer.

4. Roast the salmon and vegetables in the preheated oven for 15-20 minutes, or until the salmon is cooked through and the vegetables are tender.

5. Remove the baking sheet from the oven and drizzle the lemon juice over the salmon. Serve the salmon fillets with the roasted vegetables.

Nutritional Information (per serving, 1 salmon fillet with 1 cup roasted vegetables):
- Calories: 300
- Total Fat: 15g
- Saturated Fat: 2.5g
- Carbohydrates: 10g
- Fiber: 3g
- Protein: 30g
- Sodium: 350mg

This salmon with roasted vegetables is a great diabetic-friendly option for men. Salmon is a rich source of heart-healthy omega-3 fatty acids, while the roasted vegetables provide fiber, vitamins, and minerals. The simple seasoning and lemon juice add flavor without added sugars or excessive sodium. Adjust the portion sizes as needed to fit your individual dietary needs.

103. Turkey Burger on Lettuce Bun

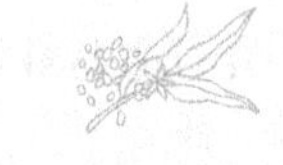

PREP TIME
20 MINUTES

COOK TIME
30 MINUTES

INGREDIENTS :

- 1 lb ground turkey
- 1/4 cup diced onion
- 1 clove garlic, minced
- 1 tsp Dijon mustard
- 1 tsp Worcestershire sauce
- 1/4 tsp salt
- 1/4 tsp black pepper
- 4 large lettuce leaves (such as romaine or iceberg)
- Toppings (optional): tomato slices, avocado, pickles, etc.

PROCEDURE :

1. In a medium bowl, combine the ground turkey, onion, garlic, Dijon mustard, Worcestershire sauce, salt, and pepper. Mix well until the ingredients are evenly distributed.

2. Divide the turkey mixture into 4 equal portions and shape them into patties, about 1/2 inch thick.

3. Preheat a grill or grill pan over medium-high heat. Cook the turkey burgers for 4-5 minutes per side, or until they are cooked through and no longer pink in the center.

4. Place each cooked turkey burger on a large lettuce leaf, using the leaf as a bun.

5. Top the burgers with your desired toppings, such as tomato slices, avocado, or pickles.

Nutritional Information (per serving, 1 turkey burger with lettuce bun):
- Calories: 200
- Total Fat: 10g
- Saturated Fat: 2.5g
- Carbohydrates: 3g
- Fiber: 1g
- Protein: 24g
- Sodium: 350mg

This turkey burger on a lettuce bun is a great diabetic-friendly option for men. The lean turkey provides a good source of protein, while the lettuce bun keeps the meal low in carbs. You can customize the toppings to your liking, adding healthy fats and additional nutrients. Adjust the portion sizes as needed to fit your individual dietary needs.

104. Veggie Stir-Fry with Tofu

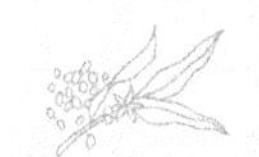

PREP TIME
20 MINUTES

COOK TIME
30 MINUTES

INGREDIENTS :

- 1 block (14 oz) extra-firm tofu, cubed
- 2 tbsp low-sodium soy sauce
- 1 tbsp rice vinegar
- 1 tsp sesame oil
- 1 tbsp olive oil
- 1 cup sliced mushrooms
- 1 cup broccoli florets
- 1 cup sliced bell peppers
- 1 cup snow peas or snap peas
- 2 cloves garlic, minced
- 1 tsp grated fresh ginger
- 2 tbsp low-sodium vegetable broth
- 1 tsp cornstarch
- Salt and pepper to taste
- Cooked brown rice, for serving (optional)

PROCEDURE :

1. In a small bowl, combine the cubed tofu, soy sauce, rice vinegar, and sesame oil. Toss to coat and set aside. Heat the olive oil in a large skillet or wok over medium-high heat.

2. Add the mushrooms, broccoli, bell peppers, and snow peas. Stir-fry for 3-4 minutes, until the vegetables are crisp-tender. Add the garlic and ginger and stir-fry for 1 minute more.

3. In a small bowl, whisk together the vegetable broth and cornstarch. Pour this mixture into the skillet and stir to coat the vegetables.

4. Add the marinated tofu and its marinade to the skillet. Stir-fry for 2-3 minutes, until the sauce has thickened slightly.

7. Season with salt and pepper to taste. Serve the veggie stir-fry over cooked brown rice, if desired.

Nutritional Information (per serving, 1 cup stir-fry without rice):
- Calories: 180
- Total Fat: 10g
- Saturated Fat: 1.5g
- Carbohydrates: 12g
- Fiber: 4g
- Protein: 14g
- Sodium: 350mg

This veggie stir-fry with tofu is a great diabetic-friendly option for men. The tofu provides a lean protein source, while the variety of vegetables add fiber, vitamins, and minerals. The stir-fry is low in carbs and calories, making it a healthy and satisfying meal. Adjust the portion sizes as needed to fit your individual dietary needs.

105. Chicken and Avocado Salad

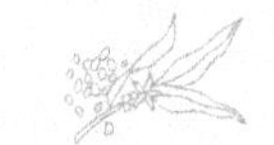

PREP TIME
20 MINUTES

COOK TIME
30 MINUTES

INGREDIENTS:

- 2 cups cooked, shredded chicken breast
- 1 ripe avocado, diced
- 1/4 cup diced red onion
- 1/4 cup diced celery
- 2 tbsp plain Greek yogurt
- 1 tbsp Dijon mustard
- 1 tbsp lemon juice
- 1/4 tsp garlic powder
- Salt and pepper to taste
- Mixed greens or lettuce leaves, for serving

PROCEDURE:

1. In a medium bowl, combine the shredded chicken, diced avocado, red onion, and celery.

2. In a small bowl, whisk together the Greek yogurt, Dijon mustard, lemon juice, and garlic powder.

3. Pour the yogurt dressing over the chicken and avocado mixture and gently toss to coat.

4. Season the salad with salt and pepper to taste.

5. Serve the chicken and avocado salad on a bed of mixed greens or lettuce leaves.

Nutritional Information (per serving, 1 cup salad):
- Calories: 220
- Total Fat: 12g
- Saturated Fat: 2g
- Carbohydrates: 6g
- Fiber: 3g
- Protein: 22g
- Sodium: 300mg

This chicken and avocado salad is a great diabetic-friendly option for men. The lean protein from the chicken, healthy fats from the avocado, and fiber from the vegetables make it a well-balanced and nutrient-dense meal. The Greek yogurt dressing provides creaminess without adding too many carbs or calories.

You can serve this salad on its own or with a side of whole grain crackers or a small portion of cooked quinoa or brown rice. Adjust the portion sizes as needed to fit your individual dietary needs.

106. Stuffed Bell Peppers with Quinoa

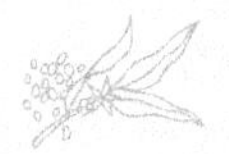
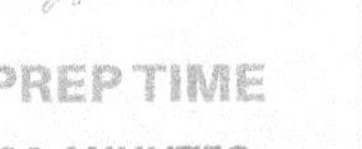
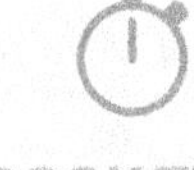

PREP TIME
20 MINUTES

COOK TIME
30 MINUTES

INGREDIENTS:

- 4 medium bell peppers (any color)
- 1 cup cooked quinoa
- 1 (15 oz) can black beans, rinsed and drained
- 1 cup diced tomatoes
- 1/2 cup shredded low-fat cheddar cheese
- 1/4 cup chopped onion
- 2 cloves garlic, minced
- 1 tsp ground cumin
- 1/4 tsp chili powder
- Salt and pepper to taste

PROCEDURE:

1. Preheat the oven to 375°F.

2. Cut the tops off the bell peppers and remove the seeds and membranes. Place the peppers in a baking dish.

3. In a medium bowl, combine the cooked quinoa, black beans, diced tomatoes, 1/4 cup of the shredded cheese, onion, garlic, cumin, chili powder, salt, and pepper. Mix well.

4. Stuff the bell pepper cavities evenly with the quinoa mixture.

5. Top the stuffed peppers with the remaining 1/4 cup of shredded cheese.

6. Bake for 25-30 minutes, or until the peppers are tender and the cheese is melted. Serve hot.

Nutritional Information (per serving, 1 stuffed pepper):
- Calories: 220
- Total Fat: 5g
- Saturated Fat: 2g
- Carbohydrates: 32g
- Fiber: 8g
- Protein: 12g
- Sodium: 400mg

These stuffed bell peppers with quinoa are a great diabetic-friendly option for men. The quinoa and black beans provide a good source of complex carbohydrates and fiber, while the bell peppers and tomatoes add important vitamins and minerals. The low-fat cheese adds a touch of creaminess without too much saturated fat. Adjust the portion sizes as needed to fit your individual dietary needs.

107. Beef and Vegetable Skewers

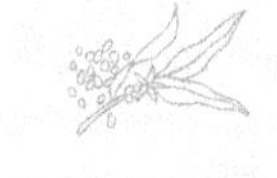 

PREP TIME
20 MINUTES

COOK TIME
30 MINUTES

INGREDIENTS :

- 1 lb beef sirloin, cut into 1-inch cubes
- 1 red bell pepper, cut into 1-inch pieces
- 1 yellow onion, cut into 1-inch pieces
- 8 oz mushrooms, halved
- 1 zucchini, cut into 1-inch pieces
- 2 tbsp olive oil
- 2 tbsp balsamic vinegar
- 1 tsp dried oregano
- 1/2 tsp garlic powder
- 1/4 tsp salt
- 1/4 tsp black pepper

PROCEDURE :

1. Preheat grill or grill pan to medium-high heat.

2. In a large bowl, combine the beef cubes, bell pepper, onion, mushrooms, and zucchini.

3. In a small bowl, whisk together the olive oil, balsamic vinegar, oregano, garlic powder, salt, and pepper.

4. Pour the marinade over the beef and vegetables and toss to coat evenly.

5. Thread the marinated beef and vegetables onto skewers, alternating the ingredients.

6. Grill the skewers for 12-15 minutes, turning occasionally, until the beef is cooked through and the vegetables are tender.

7. Serve the grilled beef and vegetable skewers immediately.

Nutritional Information (per serving, 2 skewers):
- Calories: 250
- Total Fat: 12g
- Saturated Fat: 3g
- Carbohydrates: 12g
- Fiber: 3g
- Protein: 24g
- Sodium: 300mg

These beef and vegetable skewers are a great diabetic-friendly option for men. The lean beef provides protein, while the variety of vegetables add fiber, vitamins, and minerals. The simple marinade adds flavor without excessive sodium or added sugars.

108. Grilled Tilapia with Asparagus

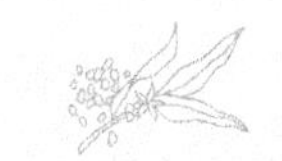 

PREP TIME
20 MINUTES

COOK TIME
30 MINUTES

INGREDIENTS :

- 4 (6 oz) tilapia fillets
- 1 tbsp olive oil
- 1 tsp lemon zest
- 1 tbsp lemon juice
- 1 tsp dried oregano
- 1/4 tsp salt
- 1/4 tsp black pepper
- 1 lb asparagus, trimmed
- 1 tbsp unsalted butter, melted

PROCEDURE :

1. Preheat grill or grill pan to medium-high heat.

2. In a small bowl, combine the olive oil, lemon zest, lemon juice, oregano, salt, and pepper. Brush this mixture evenly over both sides of the tilapia fillets.

3. Place the tilapia fillets on the preheated grill and cook for 4-5 minutes per side, or until the fish flakes easily with a fork.

4. In a large bowl, toss the asparagus spears with the melted butter.

5. Place the asparagus on the grill and cook for 5-7 minutes, turning occasionally, until tender-crisp.

6. Serve the grilled tilapia fillets with the grilled asparagus.

Nutritional Information (per serving, 1 tilapia fillet and 1/4 lb asparagus):
- Calories: 220
- Total Fat: 9g
- Saturated Fat: 3g
- Carbohydrates: 5g
- Fiber: 2g
- Protein: 30g
- Sodium: 300mg

This grilled tilapia with asparagus is a great diabetic-friendly option for men. Tilapia is a lean, mild-flavored fish that is high in protein and low in carbs. The asparagus provides fiber, vitamins, and minerals. The simple lemon and herb seasoning adds flavor without added sugars or excessive sodium.

109. Lentil and Veggie Stew

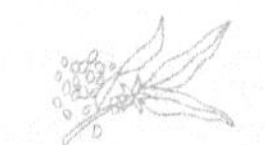

PREP TIME
20 MINUTES

COOK TIME
30 MINUTES

INGREDIENTS:

- 1 cup dry brown or green lentils, rinsed
- 4 cups low-sodium vegetable broth
- 1 tbsp olive oil
- 1 onion, diced
- 3 cloves garlic, minced
- 2 carrots, peeled and diced
- 2 celery stalks, diced
- 1 cup diced zucchini
- 1 (14.5 oz) can diced tomatoes
- 2 tsp dried thyme
- 1 tsp dried oregano
- 1/4 tsp red pepper flakes (optional)
- Salt and pepper to taste
- Chopped fresh parsley for garnish (optional)

PROCEDURE:

1. In a large pot, combine the lentils and vegetable broth. Bring to a boil over high heat.
2. Reduce heat to medium-low, cover, and simmer for 15-20 minutes, or until the lentils are tender.
3. In a separate large pot or Dutch oven, heat the olive oil over medium heat. Add the onion and sauté for 3-4 minutes until translucent.
4. Add the garlic, carrots, celery, and zucchini. Sauté for 5-7 minutes, until the vegetables are starting to soften.
5. Stir in the diced tomatoes, thyme, oregano, and red pepper flakes (if using). Season with salt and pepper.
6. Add the cooked lentils and their broth to the vegetable mixture. Stir to combine.
7. Bring the stew to a simmer and cook for 10-15 minutes, or until the vegetables are tender.
8. Serve the lentil and veggie stew hot, garnished with chopped fresh parsley if desired.

Nutritional Information (per serving, about 1 1/2 cups):
- Calories: 250
- Total Fat: 5g
- Saturated Fat: 1g
- Carbohydrates: 38g
- Fiber: 12g
- Protein: 15g
- Sodium: 350mg

This lentil and veggie stew is a great diabetic-friendly option for men. Lentils are a high-fiber, high-protein legume that can help regulate blood sugar levels. The variety of vegetables provides additional fiber, vitamins, and minerals. Adjust the portion sizes as needed to fit your individual dietary needs.

110. Stuffed Mushrooms with Turkey Sausage

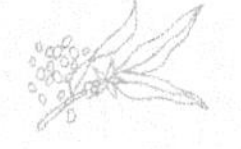 

PREP TIME
20 MINUTES

COOK TIME
30 MINUTES

INGREDIENTS :

- 24 large mushrooms, stems removed and finely chopped
- 1 lb ground turkey sausage
- 1/2 cup Italian breadcrumbs
- 1/4 cup grated Parmesan cheese
- 2 cloves garlic, minced
- 2 tbsp chopped fresh parsley
- 1/4 tsp salt
- 1/4 tsp black pepper

PROCEDURE :

1. Preheat oven to 375°F. Clean the mushrooms and remove the stems, finely chopping the stems.

2. In a skillet over medium heat, cook the turkey sausage until browned and cooked through, 5-7 minutes, breaking it up as it cooks. Drain any excess fat.

3. In a bowl, mix together the chopped mushroom stems, cooked sausage, breadcrumbs, Parmesan, garlic, parsley, salt and pepper until well combined.

4. Stuff the mushroom caps evenly with the sausage mixture, packing it in gently.

5. Arrange the stuffed mushrooms on a baking sheet. Bake for 12-15 minutes, until the mushrooms are tender and the filling is hot.

6. Serve the stuffed mushrooms warm. Enjoy!

111. Cauliflower Crust Pizza

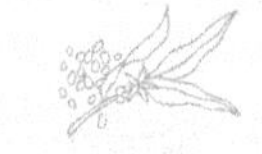

PREP TIME
20 MINUTES

COOK TIME
30 MINUTES

INGREDIENTS :

- 1 head of cauliflower, cut into florets (about 4 cups riced)
- 1 egg, lightly beaten
- 1/2 cup shredded part-skim mozzarella cheese
- 2 tbsp grated Parmesan cheese
- 1 tsp dried oregano
- 1/4 tsp garlic powder
- 1/4 tsp salt
- Toppings of your choice (such as tomato sauce, additional cheese, vegetables, etc.)

Nutritional Information (per serving, 1/4 of the pizza):
- Calories: 150
- Total Fat: 8g
- Saturated Fat: 3g
- Carbohydrates: 10g
- Fiber: 3g
- Protein: 12g
- Sodium: 400mg

PROCEDURE :

1. Preheat the oven to 400°F. Line a baking sheet with parchment paper.

2. Place the cauliflower florets in a food processor and pulse until it resembles the texture of rice or couscous.

3. Transfer the riced cauliflower to a clean kitchen towel or cheesecloth. Wring out as much moisture as possible.

4. In a medium bowl, combine the riced cauliflower, egg, mozzarella cheese, Parmesan cheese, oregano, garlic powder, and salt. Mix well until fully incorporated.

5. Press the cauliflower mixture onto the prepared baking sheet, forming a thin, even crust.

6. Bake the crust for 20-25 minutes, or until it's golden brown and cooked through.

7. Remove the crust from the oven and add your desired toppings.

8. Return the pizza to the oven and bake for an additional 10-15 minutes, or until the toppings are heated through and the cheese is melted.

9. Slice and serve the cauliflower crust pizza.

This cauliflower crust pizza is a great diabetic-friendly option for men. The cauliflower crust is low in carbs and high in fiber, while the toppings can be customized to your liking. Adjust the portion sizes and toppings as needed to fit your individual dietary needs.

112. Zucchini Fries

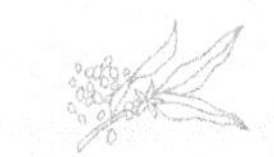 

PREP TIME
20 MINUTES

COOK TIME
30 MINUTES

INGREDIENTS :

- 2 medium zucchini, cut into 1/4-inch thick fry-shaped pieces
- 1 tbsp olive oil
- 1/4 cup grated Parmesan cheese
- 1/4 cup whole wheat breadcrumbs
- 1 tsp garlic powder
- 1/2 tsp paprika
- 1/4 tsp salt
- 1/4 tsp black pepper

Nutritional Information (per serving, about 10 fries):
- Calories: 100
- Total Fat: 5g
- Saturated Fat: 1.5g
- Carbohydrates: 10g
- Fiber: 2g
- Protein: 5g
- Sodium: 250mg

PROCEDURE :

1. Preheat the oven to 400°F. Line a baking sheet with parchment paper.

2. In a large bowl, toss the zucchini fries with the olive oil until evenly coated.

3. In a shallow bowl, mix together the Parmesan cheese, breadcrumbs, garlic powder, paprika, salt, and pepper.

4. Working in batches, dredge the zucchini fries in the breadcrumb mixture, pressing gently to help the coating adhere.

5. Arrange the breaded zucchini fries in a single layer on the prepared baking sheet.

6. Bake for 18-22 minutes, flipping halfway through, until the fries are golden brown and crispy.

7. Serve the zucchini fries hot.

These zucchini fries are a great diabetic-friendly option for men. Zucchini is a low-carb, high-fiber vegetable, and the baking method helps to keep the fries crispy without the need for frying. The Parmesan cheese and breadcrumb coating adds flavor and crunch without too many additional calories or carbs.

Serve the zucchini fries as a side dish or a healthy snack. You can also try dipping them in a low-sugar, low-fat dipping sauce, such as a Greek yogurt-based dip or a spicy mustard sauce.

113. Stuffed Peppers with Turkey

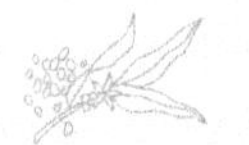 

PREP TIME
20 MINUTES

COOK TIME
30 MINUTES

INGREDIENTS :

- 6 bell peppers (any color)
- 1 lb ground turkey
- 1 cup cooked brown rice
- 1 small onion, diced
- 2 cloves garlic, minced
- 1 (14.5 oz) can diced tomatoes, no salt added
- 2 tbsp tomato paste
- 1 tsp dried oregano
- 1/2 tsp dried basil
- 1/4 tsp red pepper flakes (optional)
- 1/4 tsp salt
- 1/4 tsp black pepper
- 1/2 cup shredded low-fat mozzarella cheese

PROCEDURE :

1. Preheat oven to 375°F. Cut the tops off the peppers and remove the seeds and membranes. Place the peppers in a baking dish.

2. In a skillet over medium heat, cook the ground turkey, onion and garlic until the turkey is browned and cooked through, 5-7 minutes, breaking it up as it cooks. Drain any excess fat.

3. Stir in the cooked rice, diced tomatoes, tomato paste, oregano, basil, red pepper flakes (if using), salt and pepper. Mix well.

4. Stuff the pepper cavities evenly with the turkey-rice mixture. Top each stuffed pepper with 1-2 tbsp of the shredded mozzarella cheese.

5. Pour a small amount of water into the bottom of the baking dish. Cover the dish with foil.

6. Bake for 30-35 minutes, until the peppers are tender. Remove the foil for the last 5 minutes to allow the cheese to melt.

7. Serve the stuffed peppers warm. Enjoy!

This recipe is low in calories, carbs and fat, making it a great option for a diabetic-friendly meal. The turkey and brown rice provide protein and fiber to help keep blood sugar levels stable.

114. Chicken Lettuce Wraps

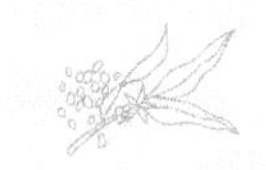

PREP TIME
20 MINUTES

COOK TIME
30 MINUTES

INGREDIENTS:

- 1 lb ground chicken or finely chopped chicken breast
- 2 tbsp sesame oil
- 3 cloves garlic, minced
- 1 tbsp grated fresh ginger
- 2 tbsp low-sodium soy sauce
- 1 tbsp rice vinegar
- 1 tbsp honey
- 1/4 tsp red pepper flakes (optional)
- 1 cup shredded carrots
- 1 cup thinly sliced mushrooms
- 1/2 cup thinly sliced green onions
- 1/4 cup chopped water chestnuts (optional)
- 12-16 large lettuce leaves (such as romaine, bibb or butter lettuce)

PROCEDURE:

1. In a large skillet or wok, cook the ground chicken over medium-high heat, breaking it up as it cooks, until no longer pink, about 5-7 minutes. Drain any excess fat.

2. Add the sesame oil, garlic and ginger to the skillet. Cook for 1 minute, stirring constantly, until fragrant.

3. Stir in the soy sauce, rice vinegar, honey and red pepper flakes (if using). Bring to a simmer and cook for 2-3 minutes.

4. Add the carrots, mushrooms, green onions and water chestnuts (if using). Cook for 2-3 minutes, until the vegetables are tender.

5. To serve, spoon the chicken mixture into the lettuce leaves. Wrap the lettuce around the filling and enjoy.

You can serve the lettuce wraps with extra soy sauce, sriracha or other desired toppings on the side. This makes a light, fresh and flavorful meal. Enjoy!

115. Veggie Burgers

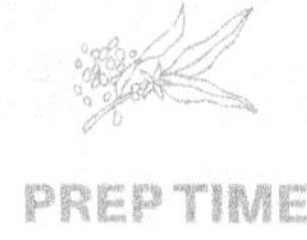

PREP TIME
20 MINUTES

COOK TIME
30 MINUTES

INGREDIENTS :

- 1 (15 oz) can black beans, rinsed and drained
- 1 cup cooked brown rice
- 1/2 cup rolled oats
- 1/2 cup finely chopped mushrooms
- 1/4 cup finely chopped onion
- 2 cloves garlic, minced
- 1 tsp chili powder
- 1/2 tsp cumin
- 1/4 tsp salt
- 1/4 tsp black pepper
- 1 egg, lightly beaten
- Whole wheat buns or lettuce leaves for serving

PROCEDURE :

1. In a large bowl, mash the black beans with a fork or potato masher until slightly chunky.

2. Add the cooked brown rice, rolled oats, mushrooms, onion, garlic, chili powder, cumin, salt and pepper. Mix well until fully combined.

3. Stir in the beaten egg until the mixture holds together.

4. Divide the mixture into 6 equal portions and shape into patties, about 1/2 inch thick.

5. Heat a large non-stick skillet over medium heat. Cook the veggie patties for 4-5 minutes per side, until lightly browned.

6. Serve the veggie burgers on whole wheat buns or wrapped in lettuce leaves. Top with your favorite condiments like mustard, avocado, tomato, etc.

These veggie burgers are high in fiber, protein and complex carbs, making them a great option for a diabetic-friendly meal. The black beans, brown rice and oats provide slow-digesting carbs to help manage blood sugar levels. Enjoy!

*As you reach the end of the **Type 1 Diabetes Cookbook for Men 110+ Recipes to Balance Blood Sugar and Satisfy Cravings,"** we hope you've found inspiration and practical solutions for managing your diabetes through delicious, satisfying meals.*

This cookbook was created with your health and enjoyment in mind. Each recipe has been carefully crafted to not only support stable blood sugar levels but also to tantalize your taste buds. From hearty breakfasts to comforting dinners and guilt-free desserts, every dish has been designed to prove that eating well with diabetes is not only possible but also enjoyable.

Beyond recipes, this book provides valuable insights into healthy eating habits tailored specifically for men. We've included tips on portion control, smart ingredient substitutions, and effective meal planning strategies to help you navigate your journey to better health with confidence.

Remember, managing diabetes is about more than just what you eat—it's about making sustainable lifestyle choices that promote long-term well-being. By incorporating the principles and recipes from this cookbook into your daily routine, you're taking proactive steps towards a healthier and more fulfilling life.

We encourage you to continue exploring new flavors, experimenting with ingredients, and discovering the joy of preparing meals that nourish both your body and your soul. With over 110 recipes at your fingertips, there's always something new to try and enjoy.

Thank you for choosing this cookbook as your guide. Here's to balanced blood sugar, satisfied cravings, and a future filled with delicious, diabetes-friendly meals. Cheers to your health and happiness!